Kazue Sawami
Wakaya Fujii
Chizuko Suishu

Development of the new preventive care for elderly and families

AF138589

Kazue Sawami
Wakaya Fujii
Chizuko Suishu

Development of the new preventive care for elderly and families

LAP LAMBERT Academic Publishing

Impressum / Imprint
Bibliografische Information der Deutschen Nationalbibliothek: Die Deutsche Nationalbibliothek verzeichnet diese Publikation in der Deutschen Nationalbibliografie; detaillierte bibliografische Daten sind im Internet über http://dnb.d-nb.de abrufbar.
Alle in diesem Buch genannten Marken und Produktnamen unterliegen warenzeichen-, marken- oder patentrechtlichem Schutz bzw. sind Warenzeichen oder eingetragene Warenzeichen der jeweiligen Inhaber. Die Wiedergabe von Marken, Produktnamen, Gebrauchsnamen, Handelsnamen, Warenbezeichnungen u.s.w. in diesem Werk berechtigt auch ohne besondere Kennzeichnung nicht zu der Annahme, dass solche Namen im Sinne der Warenzeichen- und Markenschutzgesetzgebung als frei zu betrachten wären und daher von jedermann benutzt werden dürften.

Bibliographic information published by the Deutsche Nationalbibliothek: The Deutsche Nationalbibliothek lists this publication in the Deutsche Nationalbibliografie; detailed bibliographic data are available in the Internet at http://dnb.d-nb.de.
Any brand names and product names mentioned in this book are subject to trademark, brand or patent protection and are trademarks or registered trademarks of their respective holders. The use of brand names, product names, common names, trade names, product descriptions etc. even without a particular marking in this work is in no way to be construed to mean that such names may be regarded as unrestricted in respect of trademark and brand protection legislation and could thus be used by anyone.

Coverbild / Cover image: www.ingimage.com

Verlag / Publisher:
LAP LAMBERT Academic Publishing
ist ein Imprint der / is a trademark of
OmniScriptum GmbH & Co. KG
Heinrich-Böcking-Str. 6-8, 66121 Saarbrücken, Deutschland / Germany
Email: info@lap-publishing.com

Herstellung: siehe letzte Seite /
Printed at: see last page
ISBN: 978-3-659-33316-3

Zugl. / Approved by: Kashihara, Nara, Nara Medical University, February, 2015

Preface

The evolution of an aging society is a major issue shared by economically developed countries. Among these nations, the percentage of the population aged 65 years and older is expected to hit 20–30% by the year 2050. This situation makes research on how to perceive a super-aged society where people can enjoy life to the full an absolute imperative.

In Japan, the percentage of the population aged 65 years and older is already more than 25%, making it the oldest economically developed population in the world. Japan also has the longest life expectancy in the world, with both men and women living an average of 80 years or longer. It is especially noteworthy that Japan's population is not only living longer, but also staying healthy. In 2000, a study by the World Health Organization (WHO) showed that the average Japanese person would enjoy a healthy life up to the age of 74.5 years.

In 2006, a national project to initiate long-term preventative care services began with the aim of helping Japan's elderly population maintain and elevate their physical and mental faculties for longer. The services work to assess the physical and mental faculties of the elderly, and to provide individualized preventative care. The long-term preventative care service consists of six programs: Physical Ability Improvement, Nutrition Improvement, Improvement of Oral Condition, Prevention of Cognitive Impairment, Prevention of Depression, and Housebound Solutions. It is hoped that these programs will continue to grow and develop. However, individual improvement rates following implementation of the programs and consistency in practice still pose challenges.

Our first task will be to clarify the factors that improve physical and mental function, and to promote consistency in practice. The second is the issue of Japan's family caregivers, who are also aging; for example, an elderly wife caring for her elderly husband. When the family caregivers are elderly, and there is no additional support in the immediate community, it is difficult for them to

1

obtain caregiving information and caregiver burnout tends to build up. If family caregivers are able to obtain support and acquire knowledge related to caregiving and preventative methods, the burden of caregiving can be reduced.

Through this project, we hope to provide some solutions to these issues.

Principal Investigator
Kazue Sawami

Contents

Chapter 1.   Research Overview

1. Introduction

In Japan, long-term preventative care services were introduced in 2006 as a national-scale project in order to support the wishes of Japan's elderly population to live out their lives independently for as long as possible in the community with which they are familiar. The service providers work to assess the physical and mental faculties of the elderly, and to provide individualized preventative care.

This preventative care service consists of six programs: Physical Ability Improvement, Nutrition Improvement, Improvement of Oral Condition, Prevention of Cognitive Impairment, Prevention of Depression, and Housebound Solutions.

The first step is to evaluate an individual's function based on a checklist of physical and mental faculties. A personalized preventative care program is then designed based on these results. Thereby, an elderly person can be helped to sustain and elevate their physical and mental health. With the objective of further promoting these efforts, the Ministry of Health, Labor & Welfare has recommended the development of new preventative programs. [1] The first goal of our research is to develop new preventative care programs and test them for efficacy.

Our second task is to address so-called "old-to-old caregiving," or care for the elderly by the elderly, since so many of Japan's family caregivers are themselves elderly. [2] This situation readily gives rise to caregiver burnout, which is especially likely when there is no support in the immediate community. Caregivers find it difficult to obtain information about caregiving, and feelings of isolation increase. If family caregivers are able to obtain support and acquire knowledge related to caregiving and preventative methods, the burden of caregiving can be reduced. Therefore, the second goal of our research is to develop support measures for family caregivers and test them for efficacy.

Keywords: Elderly, Family Caregivers, Mental stress, Physical & Mental Faculties, Preventative Long-Term Care

2. Physical & Mental Faculty Checklist for Preventative Long-Term Care Services

Screening by preventative long-term care services consists of an evaluation of faculties using a 25-item checklist based on Ministry of Health, Labour & Welfare guidelines (see Table 1-1). In addition to Physical Ability, Nutrition, Oral Condition, Housebound life, Forgetfulness and Depression, this checklist evaluates items related to daily life, and sets forth criteria as below. Determinations are made using the total of the values "0 or 1" shown in the answer column of Table 1-1. Responders are the subjects of the preventative long-term care services.

Table 1-1. Basic health check list for those over 65years old

NO		Questionnaire	Circle either one
daily life	1	Do you normally travel by bus or train by yourself?	0. Yes 1. No
	2	Do you go out and by daily necessities by yourself?	0. Yes 1. No
	3	Do you manage your own deposits and savings at the bank?	0. Yes 1. No
	4	Do you often go out to visit your friends?	0. Yes 1. No
	5	Do you consult with your family or friends about their	0. Yes 1. No
physical ability	6	Are you able to go upstairs without holding rail or wall?	0. Yes 1. No
	7	Are you able to stand up from the chair without any aids?	0. Yes 1. No
	8	Are you able to keep walking for about 15 minutes?	0. Yes 1. No
	9	Have you fallen during the past year?	1. Yes 0. No
	10	Do you worry about falling down?	1. Yes 0. No
nutrition	11	Have you lost more than 2~3 kg in the past 6 months?	1. Yes 0. No
	12	BMI= weight (kg) ÷ height(m)× height(m) is less than 18.5 【Height cm】【weight kg】	1. Yes 0. No
oral	13	Compared with six months ago, do you have difficulty in eating	1. Yes 0. No

condition			hard food?	
	14		Do you choke when you drink tea or soup?	1. Yes 0. No
	15		Do you often feel your mouth dry?	1. Yes 0. No
house	16		Do you go out more than once in a week?	0. Yes 1. No
bound	17		Compared with last year, do you go out less often?	1. Yes 0. No
Forgetful	18		Do people around you say you repeat the same thing and have become forgetful?	1. Yes 0. No
ness	19		Do you make phone calls by yourself?	0. Yes 1. No
	20		Do you find yourself not knowing today's date?	1. Yes 0. No
depression	21		I do not feel any fulfillment in my daily life during the last two weeks.	1. Yes 0. No
	22		I can not enjoy things I used to enjoy during the last two weeks.	1. Yes 0. No
	23		During the last two weeks, I am not willing to do what I could do easily before.	1. Yes 0. No
	24		During the last two weeks, I do not feel I am useful to anyone.	1. Yes 0. No
	25		During the last two weeks, I feel I am exhausted without any reason.	1. Yes 0. No

The source: Ministry of Health, Labour and Welfare Japan.

① Daily Life : Ten points or more for items 1-20
② Physical Ability : Three points or more for items 6-10
③ Nutrition : Items 11-12 are both applicable
④ Oral Condition : Two points or more for items 13-15
⑤ Housebound life : Item 16 is applicable, and if item 17 is applicable special
    attention is required
⑥ Forgetfulness : One point or more for items 18-20
⑦ Depression : Two points or more for items 21-25

3. **Research Method**
   ① **Pre-test 1: Relations between a subjective health and the mental and physical ability.**

In order to develop a preventative care program, we first clarified the relationship between mental and physical ability (daily life, physical ability, nutrition, oral condition, housebound, forgetfulness, depression) and subjective health (Short-form 36-item health survey version 2: SF36 v2).

Subjects: 2,000 elderly participants selected randomly from the Basic Resident Register.

Analysis: We clarified what effect subjective health had on mental and physical function using a multiple regression analysis.

② **Pre-test 2: Structural analysis of willingness to participate.**

Second, we clarified the structure of the elderly participants' willingness to participate in the preventative care project. The tools used were willingness to participate, Philadelphia Geriatric Center Morale Scale (PGC Morale Scale), the Vitality Index, and the SF36v2.

Subjects: 150 elderly participants.

Analysis: We clarified the structure of willingness to participate with a covariance structure analysis.

③ **Pre-test 3: Quality of Life of elderly people with dementia.**

Third, we clarified the factors that influence the QOL of elderly people with dementia. Through comparison of the QOL of elderly people with dementia in Japan and China and the influencing factors thereof, we extracted the characteristic determining factors among Japan's elderly people with dementia. Survey items included age, sex, personality, educational background, economic conditions, past illness, and instrumental activities of daily living (IADL), and the Dementia Quality of Life Instrument (D-QOL).

Subjects: 205 Japanese elderly people with dementia, and 187 Chinese elderly people with dementia

Analysis: A one-way analysis of variance, multiple comparisons, and a chi-square test.

④ **Pre-test 4: Mental stress of the elderly.**

Fourth, since the elderly are easily exposed to mental stress caused by experiences of loss, we clarified the effect that the amount of stress and the

7

degree of stress relief have on the subjective sense of health. The survey items included age, sex, the presence or absence and degree of stress in the preceding month, the presence or absence and degree of stress relief, and subjective sense of health.

Subjects: 40 elderly participants

Analysis: We clarified the relationship between subjective sense of health and mental stress using a Pearson product-moment correlation coefficient.

⑤ **Pre-test 5: Literature research on oral care and investigation of oral care problems.**

Fifth, we conducted literature research on improving eating and swallowing ability, and investigated the situation of people suffering from oral problems.

Subjects: 40 elderly participants

Analysis: We clarified the relationship between subjective sense of health and oral function using a Pearson product-moment correlation coefficient.

4. Creation of a preventative care program for the elderly and family caregivers

① **Fitness test of physical ability and the cognitive function of subjects.**

Conduct a physical fitness test of elderly subjects (self-check sheet, standing test, two-step test) and cognitive ability test (hand movement speed task for motor function, character position matching task for attention function, cued recall task for memory and learning ability, animal name recall task for language function, and clock drawing task for visual-spatial cognitive function) and create a preventative care program suited to the subjects' abilities.

② **Preventative Care Program.**

A 90 minute session once per month for 90 subjects, including the elderly and their families: Gather the elderly and their families, exchange information between families, and give instruction in the preventative care program: exercise, dementia prevention, stress care, eating and swallowing improvement, dietary guidance, and feedback on effectiveness.

5. Implement preventative care program for the elderly and their family caregivers and evaluate before and after the intervention.

① Physical fitness evaluation: Locomo 25, standing test, two-step test

The Locomotive Syndrome Test 25 (Locomo 25) is a test to check the subject's current mobility function in comparison to the mean for his/her age. This is a questionnaire of physical condition and living condition and is composed of 25 items.

The standing test measures leg strength by having the subject rise from a determined height using one leg or both legs.

The two-step test measures the stride of two steps to evaluate lower limb muscle strength, balance, flexibility, and other aspects of walking ability.

② Exercise behaviour change scale (SEBC)

The five stages of change are precontemplation, contemplation, preparation, action, and maintenance. Scoring was as following; precontemplation: 1 point, contemplation: 2 points, preparation: points 3, action: 4 points, and maintenance: 5 points.

③ Cognitive function evaluation: Five Cog

This measures the five cognitive functions (memory, attention, thought, language, and visual-spatial perception) that decrease with Aging-associated Cognitive Decline (AACD).

④ Self-efficacy for exercise (SEE)

This is the section which evaluates the confidence in performing exercises. The questions asks to answer out of the 5 ratings on the confidence in performing exercises when physically tired, with mental stress, when busy, and the weather is not good.

⑤ Sense of coherence (SOC)

The Japanese version of "The 13-item Sense of Coherence Questionnaire" was prepared. SOC is a concept that reflects the ability to cope with stress. SOC consists of three subordinate concepts: manageability, meaningfulness and comprehensibility.

⑥ **Measurement of psychological reaction to stress: Profile of Mood States - Brief form (POMS)**

This uses six scales, "tension," "depression," "anger," "vigor," "fatigue," and "confusion," to measure the state of feelings and emotions. There are a total of 30 question items, and subjects respond whether they experienced each item in the preceding week on a 5-level scale ranging from "not at all" to "very much."

⑦ **Health-related quality of life (QOL) measurement: WHO-QOL26 (WHO Quality of Life 26)**

This is composed of 24 times that evaluate the four areas of QOL, the physical area, the psychological area, social relations, and the environmental area, as well as two items that evaluate overall QOL, for a total of 26 items. Subjects respond to 26 items about how they felt in the past two weeks and how satisfied they were in the past two weeks on a 5-level scale: "not at all," "just a little," "somewhat," "very much," and "extremely."

⑧ **Satisfaction with the Program Conducted**

Subjects answer how satisfied they were after the intervention on a 10-level scale from "dissatisfied" to "very satisfied."

6. Method of Analysis

The comparison between before and after the intervention is clarified with a one-way analysis of variance. The relationships between each measure are evaluated for strength and degree of relevance using a multiple regression analysis.

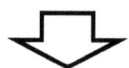

7. Program Correction

Correct the program to a highly compatible program based upon the results of the analysis.

8. Publicizing of effective program and feedback to subjects

Publicize results on the web sites of the researchers' affiliated universities and companies and through public relations brochures. Distribute the results to the subjects.

The overall flow of the entire study is depicted in Figure 1-1.

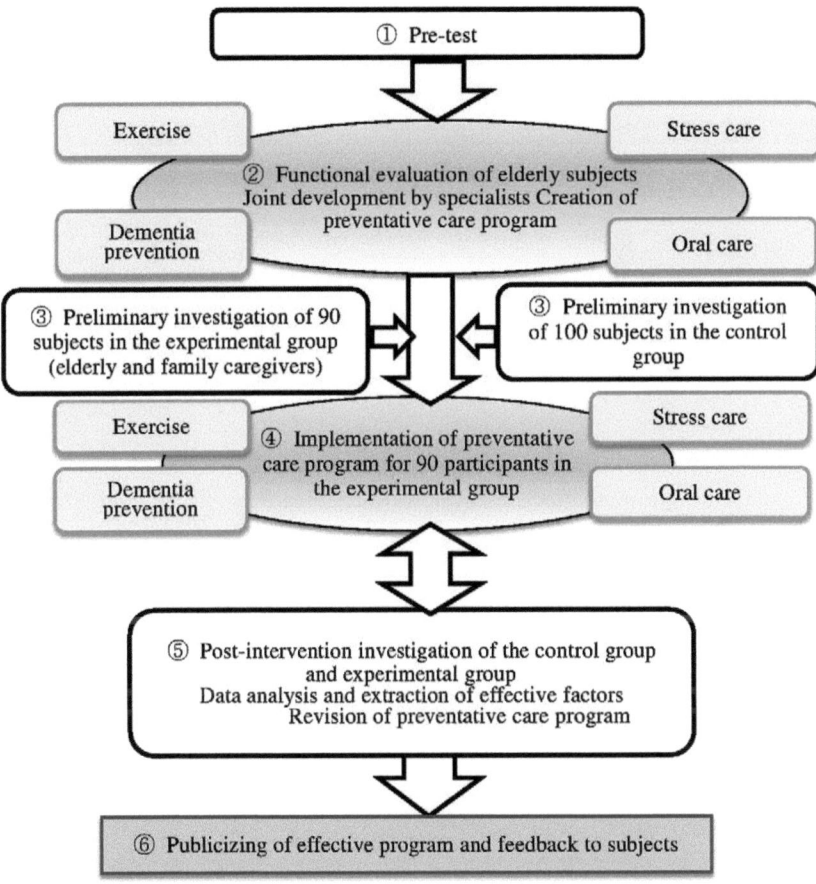

Figure 1-1. Research Flow Diagram

9. Novelty and Originality of the Research

The novelty of this research was to clarify the causal relationship of participation willingness to preventative care operations for elderly and their families, to formulate new preventive programs against care corresponding thereto, and to verify the results of intervention. In addition, a causal relationship of factors that affects body functions, cognitive functions, and QOL, was clarified. Using this result, it is aimed to improve autonomy of the subjects by predicting the future of individuals and formulating highly individualized program.

10. Ethical considerations

The outline of the research, freedom of refusal, anonymity, and details of agreement as to the publishing of results were explained to prospective participants, both in writing and verbally, and their informed consent was obtained. This study protocol was approved by the ethical review boards of institution of each researcher.

References

1) Mizuho Information & Research Institute. Report on Research & Study into the Effectiveness of the Implementation of Preventative Long-Term Care & Daily Life Support Provider Services: Elderly Rehabilitation & Health Promotion Services. 2014;20-58.
2) Cabinet Office, Government of Japan. Elder Care: 2013 Annual Report on the Aging Society. 2013;23-27.

Chapter 2.　Pre-test

Pre-test 1.
Relations between subjective health and mental and physical ability

Kazue Sawami, Naoko Morisaki, Hirofumi Hirowatari, and Hidekazu Koufuku

1.　Introduction

The goal of Japan's long-term preventative care service is to enable the elderly to acquire knowledge of preventative care measures that will help them to maintain and elevate their physical and mental health, so they will not delaying to the point of needing full-time nursing care. The subjective perception of health is related to physical and mental faculties, and is widely reported to have an impact on life expectancy in particular. [1-3] Recently, there have been reports on the relationship between the subjective perception of health and the immune system. Therefore, this is certainly a factor that should be looked at in terms of long-term preventative care. [4-6]

Long-term preventative care providers are tasked with elevating function in the areas of physical ability, nutrition, oral condition, housebound life, forgetfulness, and depression. Thus, we have clarified the relationship between these functions and the subjective perception of health using the SF-36v2 health survey. Our objective is to use this information to develop more closely targeted long-term preventative care programs. [7-8]

2.　Materials and Methods
Target population and investigation method

A total of 2000 elderly people aged 65 years or older were selected at random. They were picked out from a basic resident register randomly. Questionnaires that consisted of items from the basic health check list and the SF-36v2 were sent to them by mail.

This investigation used the following evaluation tools.

(1) Basic health check list

In the screening of the preventive care project, the target elderly population is selected using the basic health check list. This is classified into six functions: physical ability, nutrition, oral condition, housebound, forgetfulness, depression. The project participants are selected based on this result and a physiological diagnosis.

(2) SF-36v2

The SF-36v2 evaluates 36 subjective health items. This tool measures the following eight subjective health concepts; physical functioning, role physical, bodily pain, general health, social functioning, role emotional, mental health. And the independent item of the health transition.

Methods of analysis

Methods of analysis included multiple linear regression analyses (backward). The evaluating score of the basic health check list was dependent variables, and the evaluating score of the SF-36v2 was explanatory variables.

3.   Results

Questionnaires were returned from 731 people (response rate: 36.6%). Twenty-one questionnaires had missing data; therefore, 710 questionnaires were analyzed. Over half (58.6%) of the elderly people sampled had some functional decline according to the basic health check list. The basic health check list classification of 416 people with a functional decline is shown in Table 2-1.

Table 2-1. The classification of functional decline according to the basic health check list (%)

(N = 416)

Age group (y)	physical ability	oral condition	nutrition	house bound	forgetful ness	depression
60s	13.0	25.3	1.3	2.6	39.0	18.8
70s	17.9	19.9	1.5	4.1	33.1	23.5
80s	23.4	19.1	0.0	8.1	28.7	20.6
90s	26.5	11.8	0.0	11.8	14.7	35.3
Ratio across all ages	18.8	20.5	0.9	5.3	32.2	22.2

In the function classification, forgetfulness (32.2%), depression (22.2%), and oral condition (21%) showed the largest rates of functional decline. Although

14

many functions decline with aging, neither forgetfulness nor oral condition and nutrition were correlated with aging.

Table 2-2. Relationship between the basic health check list and the SF-36v2
($N = 710$)

		Function classification according to the scores of the basic health check list										
		physical ability		oral condition		nutrition		house bound		forgetful ness		depression	
		β	P	β	P	β	P	β	P	β	P	β	P
Evaluation of the SF-36v2	physical functioning	0.681	0.000	n. s.		0.172	0.018	0.225	0.003	0.254	0.002	n. s.	
	bodily pain	n. s.		n. s.		n. s.		-0.249	0.001	n. s.		n. s.	
	general health	n. s.		n. s.		0.209	0.007	0.259	0.001	0.135	0.07	0.142	0.025
	health transition	n. s.		n. s.		-0.161	0.011	-0.108	0.088	n. s.		n. s.	
	vitality	0.160	0.040	n. s.		0.177	0.036	n. s.		n. s.		0.217	0.013
	social functioning	n. s.		n. s.		0.155	0.028	0.136	0.071	0.176	0.027	n. s.	
	role emotional	n. s.		n. s.		n. s.		0.191	0.019	0.172	0.045	n. s.	
	mental health	n. s.		0.159	0.041	n. s.		n. s.		-0.131	0.104	0.212	0.005
R		0.715		0.326		0.526		0.536		0.450		0.681	
R-squared		0.511		0.106		0.277		0.287		0.202		0.464	
Adjusted R-squared		0.503		0.095		0.262		0.266		0.183		0.453	

Multiple linear regression analyses (backward); the independent scores of the basic health check list were the dependent variables.

Results of the analysis are shown on the table with standard partial regression coefficient (β), contribution ratio (R^2) and conformance of model (adjusted R^2). The β value shows the size of the impact of each independent variable (SF-36v2 score) on the dependent variable (Basic Health Check List score), where the larger the β value, the greater the impact on the dependent variant. Note that the table only includes β values with a significant variation.

It is surmised that individual factors play a large role here. The result of the multiple linear regression analysis of the basic health check list and the SF-36v2 is shown in Table 2-2.

For areas of significant relationship, subjective factors impacting Physical Ability were Physical Functioning ($\beta = 0.68$, $p < 0.01$) and Vitality ($\beta = 0.16$, p < 0.05). Subjective factors impacting Depression were General Health ($\beta = 0.14$, $p < 0.05$), Vitality ($\beta = 0.22$, $p < 0.05$) and Mental Health ($\beta = 0.21$, $p < 0.05$), and these were extracted as having a large coefficient of determination and good applicability (adjusted $R^2 > 0.45$).

We also found that Mental Health impacted Oral Condition, and Physical Functioning, General Health, Health Transition, Vitality and Social Functioning impacted Nutrition. Physical Functioning, Bodily Pain, General Health and Emotional Role impacted Housebound Life, while Physical Functioning, Social Functioning and Emotional Role impacted Forgetfulness ($\beta > 0.15$, $p < 0.05$). The coefficients of determination for these relationships were small (adjusted R^2 < 0.4), however, and probability of applicability was low.

4. Discussion

This research set out to first clarify the relationship between age and the decline in physical & mental faculties. Results showed that percentage of decline in function in Physical Ability, Housebound Life and Depression increased with age, while Oral Condition, Nutrition and Forgetfulness had no relation to age. Regarding reasons for this, it is thought that decline in Physical Ability, such as the ability to walk, manifests in a visible manner which impacts Housebound Life, in turn leading to feelings of isolation and depression, while deviation in Oral Condition and Nutrition advance silently, so that it is difficult to perceive any decline in function. Individual factors in these two areas also have a greater influence than age.

When looking at the relationship between physical & mental faculties and the subjective perception of health, which was the individual factor most focused on, Physical Ability was impacted by the subjective factors of Physical Functioning and Vitality, and applicability was at appropriate levels. When the subject perceived problems with Physical Functioning and felt a lack of Vitality, becoming unable to move around with ease was a natural outcome. For Housebound Life which increases with age, the impactful subjective factors were Bodily Pain, General Health, Physical Functioning and Emotional Role. Though applicability was low, results suggested a course of action involving a preventative program that includes pain management, an exercise approach to address Physical Functioning, and assignment of a role in life. Subjective factors impacting Depression were General Health, Vitality and Mental Health, which seems to indicate a downward spiral of poor perception of health leading to a lack of energy and deteriorating mental health. Thus, the study suggested the need for a preventative approach that can help maintain subjective perception of health.

Regarding areas that are more subject to individual factors than to the impact of aging, for Oral Condition, the impact of Mental Health was suggested although applicability was low, and the research seemed to indicate that when mental health is poor the subject does not feel like engaging in oral care. For Nutrition, relationships with Physical Functioning, General Health, Health Transition, Vitality and Social Functioning were indicated, suggesting that many subjective perceptions of health can impact nutritional status. It was thought that deterioration of nutritional status will cause all subjective perception of health factors to deteriorate, and the fact that nutritional improvement is central to long-term preventative care was verified. For Forgetfulness, relationships with Physical Functioning, Social Functioning and Emotional Role were suggested, and we were able to verify the necessity of maintaining social function and of having a role in life in order to maintain social function.

As shown above, the research clarified that subjective factors have impact on physical & mental functional expectancy which is the goal of long-term preventative care providers. Also, the importance of having a social role as an approach to social functioning was shown, in addition to approaches to physical functioning. The relationship between Activities of Daily Living and SF-36 has been clarified in studies by Martin, et al. [9], and the relationships among social roles and health-related quality of life and subjective quality of life have been clarified by Renaud, et al. [10] Our study was valuable in terms of diverting these research outcomes to the long-term preventative service providers. We would hope to develop long-term preventative programs that are appropriate to the condition and factors of the individual elderly client.

5. Conclusion

Long-term preventative care addresses Physical Ability, Nutrition, Oral Condition, Housebound Life, Forgetfulness and Depression, and the significant relationship between these functions and subjective factors has been clarified. Results also showed the importance of giving people a role in life as a social function approach, in addition to the physical function approach.

References

1) Franks P, Gold M R, and Fiscella K. Sociodemographics, self-rated health, and mortality in the US. Social Science & Medicine. 2003;56:2505-2514

2) Spiers N, Jagger C, Clarke M, et al. Are gender differences in the relationship between selfrated health and mortality enduring? Results from three birth cohorts in Melton Mowbray. United Kingdom. Gerontologist. 2003;43: 406-411.

3) Okamoto K, Tanaka Y. Subjective Usefulness and 6-Year Mortality Risks Among Elderly Persons in Japan. Gerontol B Psychol Sci Soc Sci. 2004;59:246-249.

4) Dowd JB1, Zajacova A. Does self-rated health mean the same thing across socioeconomic groups? Evidence from biomarker data. Ann Epidemiol. 2010;20:743-749.

5) Nakata A1, Takahashi M, Otsuka Y, et al. Is self-rated health associated with blood immune markers in healthy individuals? Int J Behav Med. 2010;Sep;17:234-242.

6) Tanno K, Ohsawa M, Onoda T, et al. Poor self-rated health is significantly associated with elevated C-reactive protein levels in women, but not in men, in the Japanese general population. J Psychosom Res. 2012;73:225-231.

7) Fukuhara S, Bito S, Green J, et al. Translation, adaptation, and validation of the SF-36 health survey for use in Japan. The Journal of Clinical Epidemiology 1998;51:1037-44.

8) Fukuhara S, Ware JE, Kosinski M, et al. Psychometric and clinical tests of validity of the Japanese SF-36 health survey. The Journal of Clinical Epidemiology 1998;51:1045-53.

9) Martin RL, Irrgang JJ, Burdett RG, et al. Evidence of validity for the Foot and Ankle Ability Measure (FAAM). Foot Ankle Int. 2005;26:968-983.

10) Renaud J, Levasseur M, Gresset J, et al. Health-related and subjective quality of life of older adults with visual impairment. Disability and Rehabilitation. 2010;32: 899-907.

Pre-test 2.
Structural analysis of willingness to participate

Kazue Sawami, Naoko Morisaki, Hirofumi Hirowatari, and Hidekazu Koufuku

1. Introduction

These preventative care programs aim to prevent functional decline in elderly people. The target of this project is to prevent the development of a condition that requires nursing care in 20% of the participants. However, a significant obstacle is that willingness to participate is very low, even in particularly high-risk elderly people. The target for participation was 5% of the elderly population, but less than 1% consented to participate. [1] Therefore, it is increasingly necessary for preventative care projects to promote participation in high-risk elderly people with low willingness.

Previous studies have shown a clear correlation between willingness to participate and activity and health behavior in elderly people. [2-3] Therefore, we clarified factors affecting willingness to participate and developed the participation willingness index.

2. Materials and Methods

Target population and investigation method

We measured willingness in 150 elderly people living in their own homes.

The tools that were used in this investigation were: (1) the basic health checklist; (2) the SF-36v2, to measure subjective health status; (3) the Vitality Index, to measure willingness in everyday life; (4) the Philadelphia Geriatric Center (PGC) Morale Scale, to measure subjective feelings of satisfaction; and (5) two items measuring willingness to participate in preventative care.

Newly added subjective tools

In order to establish a framework for elderly willingness to participate in preventative care, we added the following subjective tools.

Vitality Index

This tool evaluates vitality. It consists of a questionnaire that scores the following five factors: Wake Up, Communication, Feeding, On and Off Toilet, and Rehabilitation and Activity. [4]

PGC Morale Scale

This tool evaluates the morale of elderly people. It consists of three scored factors taken from a 17-item questionnaire: Agitation, Lonely Dissatisfaction, and Attitude Toward Aging. [5-6]

Two indicators of willingness to participate in preventative care

To express willingness to participate as a dependent variable, the following two items were added.

Do you want to participate in a preventative care program?   1. Yes. 2. No.

Do you think that there would be a benefit to you by participating?   1. Yes.

2. No.

Methods of Analysis

For items that were the subject of analysis, we did not use the total score of each factor's items, but simply the score of the bottom items.

We analyzed the data using correlational analysis, and covariance structure analysis, with willingness to participate in preventive care as the dependent variable, and the values of the five scales as the explanatory variables.

3.   Results

The effective answers were 121 elderly people (80.7%) with a mean ± SD age of 77± 12years. The result of subjective factors and willingness-related item had correlation. The correlation with the subjective factors and willingness-related item was shown as Table 2-3.

The strength of the relation generally according to a correlation coefficient "$0.2 \leqq r \leqq 0.4$: weak correlation, and $0.4 \leqq r$: as the strong correlation". According to this, the critical value of the factors of participation willingness was set to the correlation coefficient 0.4, and selected the items of $r > 0.4$ as effectiveness factors. The $r > 0.4$ items were extracted from items of table 1 and structured them by a structural equations modeling in the decision making of the participation. Since cronbach's alpha coefficient of these factors is high at 0.9, there is validity as an index.

Table 2-3. Correlations between subjective factors and willingness-related items (_N_ = 121)

Subjective factors		_r_
SF36v2	Current health condition	0.292**
	Healthy feeling	0.487**
	Susceptible to illness	0.417**
	Prediction of future health	0.211*
	Energetic	0.461**
	Vitality feeling	0.520**
PGC Morale Scale	Numerousness of worries	0.419**
	Fatigue	0.359**
	Susceptible to agitation	0.517**
	Insomnia by worries	0.307**
	Became irritable	0.357**
Vitality Index	Intention of communication	0.355**
Willingness to	Benefit by participating	0.567**

Pearson product-moment correlation coefficient
Criterion variables = willingness to participate in the preventative care project
*$p < 0.05$, **$p < 0.01$
Note that the table only shows items with a significant correlation.

Then, in order to clarify structure of resulting in participation, Structural Equations Modeling (SEM) was shown (Figure 2-1). The items with the high correlation with participation willingness were selected, and were shown as observable variable of SEM. Since GFI which shows the conformity of a model is 0.91, it has high validity.

As a result, the factor which has the influence strongest against decision-making of participation is "benefit by participating." This is strongly influenced by the feeling of health such as vitality and energy and the worry. In the causal relationship of structure, an improvement of these factors will raise participation willingness.

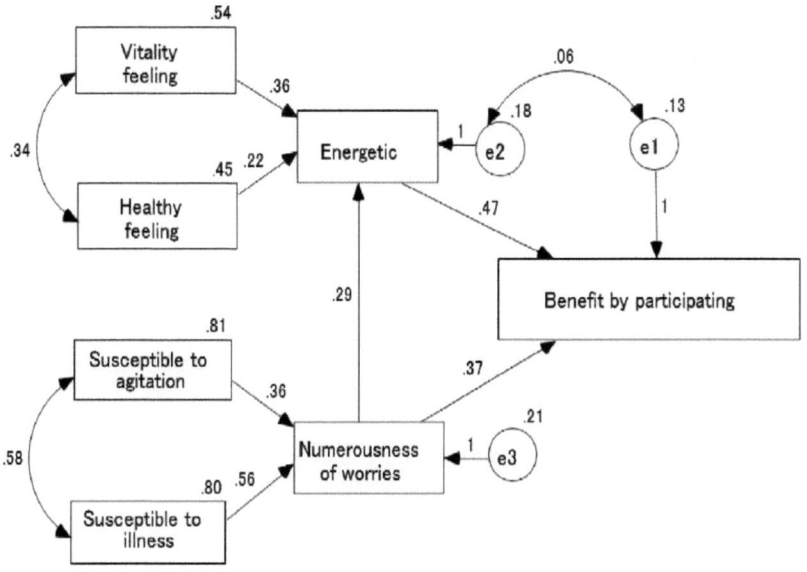

**Figure 2-1. Structural Equations Modeling
in the decision making of the participation**

About the variables of this structural model, → between observation variables is an influence index and shows the influence to the variable of the target of the arrow. ↔ is covariance and shows mutual influence. Variable e is an error variable. About these, the size of a value shows the size of influence. All the path coefficients show the significant value ($p < 0.01$).

4. Discussion

The objective of this study was to extract subjective factors that relate to Willingness to Participate in long-term preventative care projects, and to clarify the structure of elderly Willingness to Participate. As a correlation coefficient with Willingness to Participate, Benefit Of Participation was the strongest, while Feeling of Vitality and Susceptibility to Agitation had correlations of 0.5 or over. Next, Feeling of Health, Energy, Number of Worries and Susceptibility to Illness had correlations of 0.4 or over, and we used this factors to perform a structural equation modeling.

The outcome showed Energy and Number of Worries as factors directly impacting Benefit of Participation, and Number of Worries as impacting Energy. The root causes of Number of Worries were Susceptibility to Agitation and Susceptibility to Illness.

Thus, persons who do not fall ill easily and tend not to get upset, do not have many worries and are flourishing in terms of energy, and are subject to Benefit of Participation. In contrast, persons who often fall ill and are easily upset, tend to have a lot of worries and low energy, and do not readily perceive Benefit of Participation. This becomes a downward spiral where the poorer the health of the person, the less willing they are to participate in care. These outcomes are thought to suggest that these vulnerability factors can serve to inhibit the elderly from acting on behalf of their own preventative health maintenance.

Thus it may be seen that a strategy is needed to overcome the difficulty of guiding elderly persons who require intervention towards participation. Measures being implemented generally include media advertising and mobilization of transportation (fare-free), plus encouragement of participation in cultural activities, building of community networks and lifetime learning for empowerment, but these have been without major success. Efforts that have been effective at encouraging participation include personal health coaching, [7] direct mail, [8] and linking the elderly with potential sources of support, [9] and we would like to use these tactics concomitantly with measures appropriate to the structure and factors that have been clarified with this study.

Also to be considered as a distinctive psychological feature of Japan's elderly, the spouse is often perceived as the greatest support. [10] Thus, it is possible that support of the spouse is the key, and the study may indicate that participation by couples is most desirable.

5. Conclusion

The subjective factor that correlated best with Willingness to Participate was Benefit of Participating. The structural equation modeling suggested that Susceptibility to Agitation and Susceptibility to Illness as the root causes of Number of Worries were the factors that inhibited participation.

References

1) Ministry of Health, Labour & Welfare, Health & Welfare Bureau for the Elderly. Implementation Status of Secondary Preventative Service Providers: Municipalities Seminar "The Future of Long-Term Preventative Care." Ministry of Health, Labour & Welfare. 2011;7-9.

2) Grandes G, Sánchez A, Torcal J, et al. Targeting physical activity promotion in general practice: Characteristics of inactive patients and willingness to change. BMC Public Health. 2008;8:172

3) Fraenkel L, Peters E, Charpentier P, et al. Decision tool to improve the quality of care in rheumatoid arthritis. Arthritis Care Res (Hoboken). 2012;64: 977-985.

4) Toba K, Nakai R, Akishita M, et al. Vitality Index as a useful tool to assess elderly with dementia. Geriatrics & Gerontology International. 2002;2:23-29.

5) Lawton MP. Lawton's PGC MORALE SCALE. Polisher Research Institute Abramson Center for Jewish Life (formerly the Philadelphia Geriatric Center). 2003;1-9.

6) Lawton MP. The philadelphia geriatric center morale scale: a revision. Journal of Gerontology. 1975;30:85-89.

7) Cruickshank D, Tatham W Solutions for patient activation will yield the greatest benefit. Healthc Pap. 2014;13:48-53

8) Marsh AP, Lovato LC, Glynn NW, et al. Lifestyle interventions and independence for elders study: recruitment and baseline characteristics. J Gerontol A Biol Sci Med Sci. 2013;68:1549-1558.

9) Kobayashi E, Fujiwara Y, Fukaya T, et al. Social support availability and psychological well-being among the socially isolated elderly Differences by living arrangement and gender. Jpn J Public Health. 2011;58:446-456.

10) Cabinet Office, Government of Japan. Seventh International Comparison Survey of Daily Living and Awareness of the Elderly. Cabinet Office, Government of Japan. 2010;67-71.

Pre-test 3.

Quality of Life of elderly people with dementia

Chizuko Suishu, Sonomi Hattori, Tomoko Ishitani,
Xiao-Jing Li, and Feng-Lan Lou

1. Introduction

According to the 2013 World Alzheimer Report, the number of dementia patients is increasing exponentially, with an estimated 44 million at present expected to triple by the year 2050. [1] The prevalence of pre-dementia phase mild cognitive impairment (MCI) is between 16%-20% in most countries, although there are major disparities among nations as well as a number of different diagnostic standards. [2]

The rapid doubling of the prevalence rate makes planning for dementia strategy a massive and urgent challenge. In preparation for developing a program of measures against dementia, we extracted some factors related to the quality of life of elderly dementia patients, with the hope of developing a program appropriate to this population.

Health professionals need to maintain the comfort and quality of life (QOL) of cognitively impaired elderly persons, whose numbers are increasing rapidly, and their families. Therefore, we examined the subjective QOL of such persons in Japan and China, and extracted its characteristics.

2. Materials and methods

Target population and investigation method

Subjects were adults (205 Japanese, 187 Chinese) with dementia aged ≥65 years, scoring 23–15 on the Mini Mental State Examination.

Survey items included age, sex, personality, educational background, economic conditions, past illness, and instrumental activities of daily living (IADL), and the Dementia Quality of Life Instrument (D-QOL).

Methods of analysis

We conducted a one-way analysis of variance, and multiple comparisons.

3. Result

The mean age of the Japanese men (n = 37) was 84.3 ± 8.6 years, Japanese women (n = 168) was 85.7 ± 6.5 years, Chinese men (n = 81) was 77.0 ± 6.7 years, and Chinese women (n = 106) was 79.9 ± 6.8 years.

Mean D-QOL scores of the Japanese and Chinese were 118.3 ± 14.6 and 90.1 ± 15.2, respectively. Japanese D-QOL scores differed significantly by IADL functioning, educational background, and personality; Chinese scores, by past illness and economic condition.

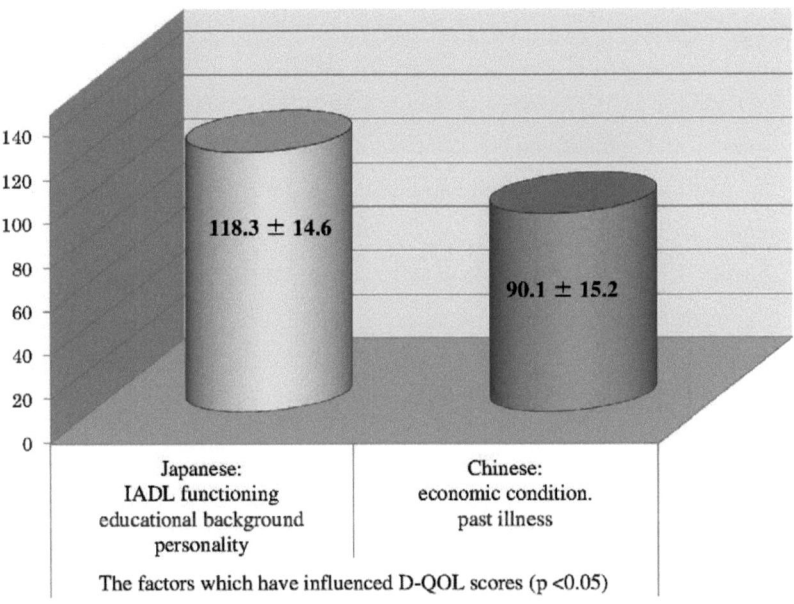

The factors which have influenced D-QOL scores (p <0.05)

Figure 2-2. D-QOL scores of the Japanese and Chinese

4. Discussion

Japanese D-QOL scores differed significantly by IADL functioning, educational background, and personality. For this reason, in Japan, functional training, lifelong learning, and enhancement of personal dignity are necessary to maintain QOL of elderly dementia patients.

These factors are consistent with the value set of Japan's elderly population, who feel that they want to perform activities of daily life under their own power. In research by Nitta, et al., abilities in exercise and social activities all impact the subjective perception of health. [3]

In Japan, municipalities are sponsoring lifelong learning for the elderly population, and together with lecture programs sponsored by universities and businesses, the number of facilities is growing year by year, but the rate of participation is not high. [4] Since this is a factor that can influence quality of life, it would seem that efforts are needed to stimulate participation.

Chinese D-QOL scores differed significantly by past illness and economic condition. For this reason, in China, preventive strategies and sufficient medical care with no additional cost are necessary for the same.

In China, it is difficult to construct a social welfare system based on a nationally unified standard, due to disparities in access to medical care and in health status. The resolution of this problem would seem to be a priority task for dementia quality of life (D-QOL). [5]

5. Conclusion

In Japan, lifelong learning, functional training, and enhancement of personal dignity are necessary to maintain QOL of elderly dementia patients. In China, preventive strategies and sufficient medical care with no additional cost are necessary for the same.

This study is the text version of the abstract that won Best Poster Award at the Singapore Health & Biomedical Congress 2013.

References

1) Alzheimer's Disease International. The global voice on dementia. The Global Impact of Dementia 2013–2050. Alzheimer's Disease International London.

2013;2-7.

2) Roberts R, Knopman DS. Classification and Epidemiology of MCI. Clin Geriatr Med. 2013;29:1-19.

3) Nitta A, Nakao R, Kawasaki R, et al. Factors influencing public health efforts in preventing life-style related illnesses and minimizing care needs among the elderly —from the perspectives of gender difference and self-rated health—. Nagasaki University's Bulletin: Health science research. 2011;23:1-8.

4) Ezawa K. The Challenge of Supporting Learning for the Elderly in the Super-Aging Society. Reference.2013;1-33.

5) Menga Q, Zhangb J, Yanc F, et al. One country, two worlds – The health disparity in China. Global public health. 2012;7:124-136.

Pre-test 4.
Mental stress of the elderly

Kazue Sawami, Naoko Morisaki, Hirofumi Hirowatari, and Hidekazu Koufuku

1. Introduction

Subjective health of the elderly may significantly influence their prognosis of life. Clinical studies are constantly carried out to determine the factors that may affect life prognosis. Among these factors is the increased susceptibility of the elderly to stress. As people age, they encounter various stressors, including the death of a family member or a friend, loss of social role by retirement, and mounting health problems. Such stress could adversely affect the subjective health of the elderly. [1-2]

Therefore, this study clarifies the degree of stress and the degree of relaxation and their association with subjective health among older adults.

2. Materials and Methods
Target population and investigation method

A questionnaire survey was administered to 40 participants in a health seminar for elderly people. Survey items were age, sex, existence of stress for the past month, stress level (five levels), relaxation degree of stress management, and subjective health for the past month.

Methods of analysis

The Pearson product-moment correlation coefficient was used for analysis.

3. Results

The respondents were 36 elderly people (90%) with a mean ± SD age of 75.5 ± 10.5 years. The sex ratio was 1:1.

Women experienced higher levels of stress than men (Table 2-4), but stress levels did not significantly differ across ages.

Table 2-4. Stress levels $N = 36$

		Stress level					
		1.None	2.Little	3.Moderat	4.Substantial	5.Unbearable	Total
Men	n	3	11	4	0	0	18
	%	16.7%	61.1%	22.2%	.0%	.0%	100.0%
Women	n	2	5	6	4	1	18
	%	11.1%	27.8%	33.3%	22.2%	5.6%	100.0%

Women showed a lower degree of relaxation than did men (Table 2-5). They reported encountering various types of stress, which were particularly felt when they were not relaxed.

Table 2-5. Relaxation degree $N = 36$

		Relaxation degree					
		1.Completely relaxed	2.Almost fully relaxed	3.Neither relaxed nor tense	4.Somewhat tensed	5.Highly tensed	Total
Men	n	9	4	4	1	0	18
	%	50.0%	22.2%	22.2%	5.6%	.0%	100.0%
Women	n	5	2	8	3	0	18
	%	27.8%	11.1%	44.4%	16.7%	.0%	100.0%

The subjective health of the elderly is shown in Table 2-6. Subjective health appeared to be lower in women than in men.

Table 2-6. Subjective health $N = 36$

		Grade of the subjective health					
		1. Excellent	2. Good	3.Neither good nor bad	4. Poor	5. Terrible	Total
Men	n	6	6	5	1	0	18
	%	33.3%	33.3%	27.8%	5.6%	.0%	100.0%
Women	n	4	3	7	3	1	18
	%	22.2%	16.7%	38.9%	16.7%	5.6%	100.0%

Subjective health was strongly correlated with both stress level (r = 0.76) and the degree of relaxation (r = 0.88). Relaxation influenced subjective health more strongly than did stress.

4. Discussion

The results show that stress influences the subjective health of the elderly; additionally, the degree of relaxation has a stronger influence on subjective health. It is therefore suggested that alleviating stress may greatly improve subjective health in this age group. To improve the subjective health of the elderly, relaxation techniques should be promoted. However, most elderly women feel that alleviation of stress is not possible. External support for stress that cannot be self-managed is necessary.

Chronic stress in elderly people deteriorates their health, and the effect of such is even stronger than that of a contagious disease. [3] In addition, relaxation is thought to improve functional ability. [4] However, few studies have examined measures to promote stress management thus far. [5] The present study aims to determine the common factors of stress in elderly women. Common stressors are revealed, and specific interventions that target these stressors should be considered. At present, the identified stressors in the elderly include age-related changes and their current health condition. [6]

While preventive care tailored to older adults has been developed, most of them have limited knowledge about stress management. The stress they experience may be possibly eased by disseminating relevant information about stress and health. However, since with decreasing interaction and social participation among senior citizens, dissemination of such knowledge is difficult. [7] More opportunities for social interaction should be provided to this age group.

5. Conclusion

The degree of mitigation of psychological stress strongly impacted the subjective perception of health. In particular, the psychological stress level of elderly women was higher that than of elderly men. Going forward, it is necessary to construct means of care for stress that cannot be resolved on one's own.

References

1) Levy BR, Hausdorff JM, Hencke R, et al. Reducing Cardiovascular Stress With Positive Self- Stereotypes of Aging. J Gerontol B Psychol Sci Soc Sci. 2000;55:205-213.

2) Kudielka BM, Buske-Kirschbaum A, Hellhammer DH, et al. HPA Axis Responses to Laboratory Psychosocial Stress in Healthy Elderly Adults, Younger Adults, and Children: Impact of Age and Gender. Psychoneuroendocrinology. 2004;29:83-98.

3) Vedhara K, Cox NK, Wilcock GK, et al. Chronic Stress in Elderly Carers of Dementia Patients and Antibody Response to Influenza Vaccination. Lancet. 1999;353:627-631.

4) Luskin F, Reitz M, Newell K, et al. A Controlled Pilot Study of Stress Management Training of Elderly Patients With Congestive Heart Failure. Prev Cardiol. 2002;5:168-172.

5) Kim E, Tsuda A, Terumi M, et al. Recent Trends in Preventive Stress Management in Japan. Kurume University Psychological Research. 2011;10:164-75.

6) Shimoyama Y, and Kanemitsu Y. Study on Stressors and Coping Behaviors of Elderly People: Based on Interviews with the Elderly People of Manabe Island. Kawasaki Medical Welfare Journal. 2005;14:267-275.

7) Ministry of Health, Labour and Welfare. Annual Health, Labour and Welfare Report. Gyosei, Tokyo. 2003;5-18.

Literature review on oral care and investigation of oral care problems

Kazue Sawami, Naoko Morisaki, and Hiroko Miura

1. Introduction

Death from pneumonia among Japan's elderly population is increasing, and in 2013 pneumonia was the 3rd leading cause of death. [1] The cause of pneumonia among the elderly is pulmonary aspiration, and what is most needed is effective preventative long-term care. Thus the objective of this study is the preparation of a preventative program for aspiration pneumonia.

First, we reviewed means for effectively preventing aspiration. The main aim of this study was to identify methods that could be easily practiced by elderly individuals. We further investigated the risk of aspiration in elderly people. The causes of aspiration include the use of dentures, [2-4] untreated periodontosis, [5-7] and dysfunctional motility of the oral cavity organs. [8-9]

Based on this information, we studied issues involving the health of the oral cavity among the elderly.

2. Materials and Methods

First, a review was conducted of the treatments for swallowing, as reported in the literature
published from 2009 to 2013. PubMed Central, BioMed Central, and InCites Journal Citation Reports were searched for relevant articles. The search terms used were "elderly people," "oral care," and "swallowing care." Articles that addressed specific oral care techniques were selected. To be included in this review, the articles had to satisfy the following requirements:
1. Methods that did not require any special apparatus
2. Methods that elderly people could practice easily at home

Next, a questionnaire regarding the oral cavity function was administered to individuals who were members of a society for elderly people. The questions addressed the following:

1. Denture use
2. Condition of the dentures
3. Details of dental examinations
4. Tough to chewing.
5. A feeling of bad condition of the oral cavity

Methods of analysis

Using Pearson's product-moment correlation coefficient, we set criterion variables of "A feeling of bad condition of the oral cavity," and looked for correlation with other items.

3. Results

We extracted 583 articles that had been published between 2009 and 2013, using the search terms "elderly people," "oral care," and "swallowing care." Eighty-five of these articles fulfilled the selection criteria and were included in the analysis (Table 2-7).

With regard to medication use, a chlorhexidine mouth rinse was reported in the most number of articles, followed by catechin gel and pneumococcal vaccine inoculation. With regard to training, most studies reported training the tongue and the oral muscles, followed by ice massage of the oral cavity. With regard to oral care, most studies reported care by a professional, followed by denture management.

An approach among these that is a possibility for self-care is to instruct the elderly subject and family members in methods of oral cavity care and therapy. In preparation for this approach we checked on issues of oral cavity function presently existing among the elderly.

The effective answers were 36 elderly people (90.0%) with a mean ± SD age of 71 ± 8.2 years. 52.8% are denture wearers, 16.7% of them feel their dentures do not fit very well. 47.2% feel a problem in their mouth either all the time or sometimes, 25.0% have trouble chewing something hard, and 61.1% were not getting dental check-ups.

Table 2-7. The aspiration prevention program to be practiced by elderly people

Method	Materials	Effect	Number of articles
Medication	Chlorhexidine mouth rinse	Plaque removal	12
	Pneumococcal vaccine inoculation	Prevention of pneumonia	4
	Catechin gel	Decrease in the growth of oral bacteria and *Candida*	4
	Moisturizer	Improved swallowing and chewing	2
	Capsaicin film use	Increased quantity of substance P in the saliva	1
	Chlorhexidine and cetylpyridinium chloride	Plaque removal	1
	Aqueous colloidal bismuth oxide nanoparticles	Plaque removal	1
	Brushing with baking soda toothpaste	Plaque removal	1
	Gargling with 3% povidone-iodine after tooth brushing	Decrease in the growth of oral bacteria and *Candida*	1
	Provision of thickener use instructions to the family	Prevention of aspiration	1
Training	Training of the tongue and oral muscles	Improved swallowing and chewing	21
	Ice massage of the oral cavity	Improved swallowing and chewing	4
	Respiratory physiotherapy	Removal of phlegm	3
Oral care	Oral care by a professional	Decrease in disease-causing germs	22
	Management of dentures	Improved swallowing and chewing	3
	Provision of oral care-related instructions to elderly people	Improved oral health-related quality of life, Plaque removal	3

For these issues that involve oral cavity function, we set "bad condition of the oral cavity" as criterion variable and tested for correlation. As shown in Table 2-8, the strongest correlation was ill-fitting dentures and pain or difficulty when chewing ($p < 0.05$).

Table 2-8. Correlation of Intra-Oral Cavity Bad Condition with
Related Factors   N=36

Oral Cavity Function Related Factors	r
Uses Dentures	.226
Ill-fitting Dentures	.473**
Pain or Difficulty Chewing	.353*
Dental Check-ups	.273

Pearson product-moment correlation coefficient
Criterion variables = A feeling of bad condition of the oral cavity.
*p<0.05, **p<0.01

There was no correlation however with dental check-ups, and subjects did not have check-ups at the dentist even when feeling bad conditions. We then looked for correlation with other factors to see under what conditions subjects would get dental check-ups, but there was no relationship with any factor (p > 0.05).

Thus, it was shown that subjects did not get dental check-ups even with ill-fitting dentures or pain or difficulty with chewing (Table 2-9).

Table 2-9. Correlation of Dental Check-ups with
Intra-Oral Cavity Problems   N=36

Oral Cavity Function Related Factors	r
Uses Dentures	-.159
Denture Fit	.255
Pain or Difficulty Chewing	-.066
Discrepancy	.273

Pearson product-moment correlation coefficient
Criterion variables = dental examinations

4. Discussion

With regard to preventive measures against aspiration, the ability of elderly people to practice these measures easily and regularly is most important. Considering the results presented in Table 1, inexpensive medicines that can be used easily and safely can be recommended. Although the validity of the chlorhexidine mouth rinse has been widely verified, it is preferable to use a gel formulation in order to allow accumulation of the agent in the mouth and additionally reduce the risk of aspiration.

Next, regarding oral care by a specialist, although most literature proves the effectiveness of receiving specialist oral care, as this study clearly showed the reality is that the elderly are not getting specialist check-ups even when they are experiencing bad oral cavity condition or ill-fitting dentures, and low priority is given to oral health. Similar reports on this subject can be found. [10-11] When self-care is given low priority, in many cases it is not practiced at all.

Even if elderly people are aware of their symptoms, they do not undergo medical examinations. Because decline in oral function does not present with symptoms, the frequency of medical examinations is low; however, even individuals who were aware of such decline tended to take their condition lightly. Therefore, it would be more useful to disseminate information regarding effective methods for preventing aspiration than to persuade participation in medical examinations.

Therefore, the dissemination of information that raises health literacy is important to ensure self-determination. For example, oral health through self-care is not widely propagated, and most articles discuss expert care. Professional care is available to a limited number of individuals and cannot be made widely available. Therefore, self-care should be widely propagated. The death rates associated with aspiration-related pneumonia will not decrease if such measures are not undertaken. The problem has been the low rate of common knowledge regarding the effectiveness of oral cavity function therapy for the prevention of pulmonary aspiration, although its effectiveness has been widely proven. [12-13] Also, it would seem that continuity of therapy for elderly living at home will be difficult if subjects or family members are not instructed in therapy that they can do themselves. We need to address both of these points with a program that can be easily disseminated. This study has shown the necessity of disseminating rapid response measures since 47.2% of elderly living at home are experiencing some kind of bad oral cavity condition.

5. Conclusion

About half of the subjects were experiencing poor oral health condition either all the time or part of the time, but there was no correlation with dental check-ups. Since it appears that oral health is of low priority, methods for effective oral cavity self-care and oral cavity therapy programs that can be done easily by the elderly person or the family need to be disseminated.

References

1) Statistics and information department, minister's secretariat, ministry of health, labour and welfare. Vital statistics in Japan. Ministry of Health, Labour and Welfare. 2014;16-23.

2) Son D S, Seong J W, Kim Y, et al. The Effects of Removable Denture on Swallowing. Ann Rehabil Med. 2013;37:247-253.

3) Monaco A, Cattaneo R, Masci C, et al. Effect of ill-fitting dentures on the swallowing duration in patients using polygraphy. 2012;29:e637-44.

4) Gilbert GH, Meng X, Duncan RP, et al. Incidence of tooth loss and prosthodontic dental care: effect on chewing difficulty onset, a component of oral health-related quality of life. J Am Geriatr Soc. 2004;52:880-885.

5) Liantonio J, Salzman B, Snyderman D. Preventing Aspiration Pneumonia by Addressing Three Key Risk Factors: Dysphagia, Poor Oral Hygiene, and Medication Use. Case Reports in Medicine. 2013;1-4.

6) Brito F, Zaltman C , Carvalho AT, et al. Subgingival microflora in inflammatory bowel disease patients with untreated periodontitis. Eur J Gastroenterol Hepatol. 2013;25:239-245.

7) Gomes-Filho I S, Passos J S, and da Cruz S S. Systemic disease and oral bacteria. Journal of Oral Microbiology. 2010; Open Access article, DOI: 10.3402/jom.v2i0.5811.

8) Ramsey D, Smithard D, and Kalra L. Silent aspiration: what do we know? Dysphagia. 2005;20: 218-225.

9) Iida T, Tohara H, Wada S, et al. Aging Decreases the Strength of Suprahyoid

Muscles Involved in Swallowing Movements. Tohoku J. Exp. Med. 2013;231:223-228.

10) Clovis JB, Brillant MG, Matthews DC, et al. Using interviews to construct and disseminate knowledge of oral health policy. Int J Dent Hyg. 2012;10:91-97.

11) Hallberg U, and Klingberg G. Giving low priority to oral health care. Voices from people with disabilities in a grounded theory study. Acta Odontol Scand. 2007;65:265-270.

12) Nakayama T. Inquiring survey of the elderly people at nursing home and their feeding condition. Niigata dental journal. 2013;43:31-39.

13) Young B C, Murray C A and Thomson J. Care home staff knowledge of oral care compared to best practice: a West of Scotland pilot study. British Dental Journal. 2008; Open Access article, DOI : 10.1038/sj.bdj.2008.894.

Chapter 3.   Creation of a preventative care program for the elderly and family caregivers

Kazue Sawami, Wakaya Fujii, Chizuko Suishu,
Katahata Yukari, and Hirofumi Hirowatari

1.   Introduction

Based on the results of the present state analysis in the previous section, we created a preventative long-term care program. Preventative long-term care programs must be suited to the immediate conditions and the needs of the subject, since these programs require consistent practice by the subject. Results of the study in the previous section showed that there is a significant relationship between the perception of subjective health and the physical and mental functions which are addressed by preventative long-term care services. Further, the subjective perception of health, which has the most powerful impact on participation in preventative long-term care services, will benefit from participation, while susceptibility to illness and anxiety were disincentive to participation. Thus in the vicinity of preventative intervention measures, we attempted to implement more precise testing of subjective health and physical & mental faculties in order to enhance the precision of preventative long-term care programs.

As stated in the previous section, Japan's elderly are characteristically reliant upon spouses for emotional support, so we devised programs in which spouses or family members can participate. We implemented preventative long-term care intervention for the elderly and instructed family members on preventative long-term care methods.

Our preventative long-term care programs consisted chiefly of interventions in exercise, mental stress care, dementia strategy and oral care. Since there was no need to improve the nutritive intake based on the physical condition of the subjects, we simply conducted a talk about nutrition without taking any intervention action.

2. Materials and Methods

A total of 100 elderly persons and family members were recruited. 90 subjects responding to the recruitment were chosen as the experimental group, physical strength and cognitive function were tested, and preventative long-term care programs suited to their faculties were devised.

Intervention to experimental group

① Fitness test of physical ability and the cognitive function of subjects.

Conduct a physical fitness test of elderly subjects (self-check sheet, standing test, two-step test) and cognitive ability test (hand movement speed task for motor function, character position matching task for attention function, cued recall task for memory and learning ability, animal name recall task for language function, and clock drawing task for visual-spatial cognitive function) and create a preventative care program suited to the subjects' abilities.

Physical fitness test

A subjective evaluation was conducted on exercise function by a self-check-sheet (table 3-1) consisting of 25 questionnaires which is supported by the Japanese Orthopedic Association and used in many places in Japan. [1]

Table 3-1. The 25-question Geriatric Locomotive Function Scale

The following questions are asking about your health status and usual daily life, relating to involvement of your back and limbs. Please answer on your status 'over the last one month'. Please check the box for the most suitable response to each question.

■ Following are questions about your body pain for the last one month:

1. Did you have any pain (including numbness) in your neck or upper limbs (shoulder, arm, or hand)?

□ No pain   □ Mild pain   □ Moderate pain   □ Considerable pain   □ Severe pain

2. Did you have any pain in your back, lower back or buttocks?

□ No pain   □ Mild pain   □ Moderate pain   □ Considerable pain   □ Severe pain

3. Did you have any pain (including numbness) in your lower limbs (hip, thigh, knee, calf, shin, ankle, ￨

□ No pain   □ Mild pain   □ Moderate pain   □ Considerable pain   □ Severe pain

42

4. To what extent has it been painful to move your body in daily life?

□ No pain   □ Mild pain   □ Moderate pain   □ Considerable pain   □ Severe pain

■Following are questions about your usual daily life for the last one month:

5.   To what extent has it been difficult to get up from a bed or lie down?

□ Not difficult   □ Mildly difficult   □ Moderately difficult   □ Considerably difficult   □ Extremely difficult

6. To what extent has it been difficult to stand up from a chair?

□ Not difficult   □ Mildly difficult   □ Moderately difficult   □ Considerably difficult   □ Extremely difficult

7. To what extent has it been difficult to walk inside the house?

□ Not difficult   □ Mildly difficult   □ Moderately difficult   □ Considerably difficult   □ Extremely difficult

8. To what extent has it been difficult to put on and take off shirts?

□ Not difficult   □ Mildly difficult   □ Moderately difficult   □ Considerably difficult   □ Extremely difficult

9. To what extent has it been difficult to put on and take off trousers and pants?

□ Not difficult   □ Mildly difficult   □Moderately difficult   □ Considerably difficult   □ Extremely difficult

10. To what extent has it been difficult to use the toilet?

□ Not difficult   □ Mildly difficult   □ Moderately difficult   □ Considerably difficult   □ Extremely difficult

11. To what extent has it been difficult to wash your body in the bath?

□ Not difficult   □ Mildly difficult   □ Moderately difficult   □ Considerably difficult   □ Extremely difficult

12. To what extent has it been difficult to go up and down stairs?

□ Not difficult   □ Mildly difficult   □ Moderately difficult   □ Considerably difficult   □ Extremely difficult

13. To what extent has it been difficult to walk briskly?

□ Not difficult   □ Mildly difficult   □ Moderately difficult   □ Considerably difficult   □ Extremely difficult

14. To what extent has it been difficult to keep yourself neat?

□ Not difficult   □ Mildly difficult   □ Moderately difficult   □ Considerably difficult   □ Extremely difficult

15. How far can you keep walking without rest? (please select the closest answer)

□ More than 2-3 km   □ approximately 1 km   □approximately 300 m   □ approximately 100 m   □ approximately 10 m

43

16. To what extent has it been difficult to go out to visit neighbors?

□ Not difficult   □ Mildly difficult   □ Moderately difficult   □ Considerably difficult   □ Extremely difficult

17. To what extent has it been difficult to carry objects weighing approximately 2 kilograms (2 standard milk bottles or 2 PET bottles each containing 1 liter)?

□ Not difficult   □ Mildly difficult   □ Moderately difficult   □ Considerably difficult   □ Extremely difficult

18. To what extent has it been difficult to go out using public transportation?

□ Not difficult   □ Mildly difficult   □ Moderately difficult   □ Considerably difficult   □ Extremely difficult

19. To what extent have simple tasks and housework (preparing meals, cleaning up, etc.) been difficult?

□ Not difficult   □ Mildly difficult   □ Moderately difficult   □ Considerably difficult   □ Extremely difficult

20. To what extent have load-bearing tasks and housework (cleaning the yard, carrying heavy bedding, etc.) been difficult?

□ Not difficult   □ Mildly difficult   □ Moderately difficult   □ Considerably difficult   □ Extremely difficult

21. To what extent has it been difficult to perform sports activity (jogging, swimming, gate ball, dancing, etc.)?

□ Not difficult   □ Mildly difficult   □ Moderately difficult   □ Considerably difficult   □ Extremely difficult

22. Have you been restricted from meeting your friends?

□ Not restricted   □ Slightly restricted   □ Restricted about half the time   □ Considerably restricted   □ Gave up all activities

23. Have you been restricted from joining social activities (meeting friends, playing sport, engaging in activities and hobbies, etc.)?

□ Not restricted   □ Slightly restricted   □ Restricted about half the time   □ Considerably restricted   □ Gave up all activities

24. Have you ever felt anxious about falls in your house?

□ Have not felt anxious   □ Have occasionally felt anxious   □ Have sometimes felt anxious   □ Have often felt anxious

□ Have constantly felt anxious

25. Have you ever felt anxious about being unable to walk in the future?

□ Have not felt anxious   □ Have occasionally felt anxious   □ Have sometimes felt anxious   □ Have often felt anxious

□ Have constantly felt anxious

The source: Atsushi Seichi, et al. Development of a screening tool for risk of locomotive syndrome in the elderly: the 25-question Geriatric Locomotive Function Scale. Journal of Orthopaedic Science. 2011

This is a survey sheet created to find disabilities in Musculoskeletal at early stages by questioning difficulties in everyday activities through 25 questions. Total of 0 points after 25 questions show the best state, 100 points as the worst state and the cut-off is 16 points.

Standing test and two step test was used as an objective evaluation of exercise function. The standing test was conducted by having the target sit on boxes of 30, 20, and 10 cm to see down to which height they can stand up with one foot, without using arms or reactions. This is deeply related to WBI (weight bearing index), knee extension muscular strength subtracted by weight, The knee extension muscular strength needed to walk is 20 cm by the standing up test while 0.45 in WBI, standing up from 40 cm by one foot is equal to 0.6 in WBI. [2-3]

In the two-step test, the subject is asked to stand with both feet together, take two steps as large as possible, and then subtract the height from the distance walked. This is said to reflect the level of self-support in daily life and the risk of falling down. The average values for a Japanese at each age is given in table 3-2 and 3-3 (The source: Japan Locomo Challenge Promotion Conference). If the subject does not meet the average value of their age, if the situation does not change, there is high possibility of disabilities to be seen in activities like walking.

Table 3-2. The mean standing test results for Japanese participants

Age (years)	Men	Women
20 – 29	20 cm*	30 cm*
30 – 39	30 cm*	40 cm*
40 – 49	40 cm*	40 cm*
50 – 59	40 cm*	40 cm*
60 – 69	40 cm*	40 cm*
70 – 79	10 cm**	10 cm**

Participants of all ages began the standing test by performing the one-leg standing test; participants who were unable to perform this test began with the two-leg standing test.
*one-leg standing test results, **two-leg standing test results

Table 3-3. The mean of the Japanese two-step test

Age	Men	Women
20－29	1.64～1.73	1.56～1.68
30－39	1.61～1.68	1.51～1.58
40－49	1.54～1.62	1.49～1.57
50 – 59	1.56～1.61	1.48～1.55
60 – 69	1.53～1.58	1.45～1.52
70 – 79	1.42～1.52	1.36～1.48

The source: Japan Locomo Challenge Promotion Conference.

The tool used for cognitive ability test is Five Cognitive Functions (Five Cog). This is made to measure the functions of 5 cognitive domains, and consists of the clock drawing task (visuospatial function), position judgment task (attention), animal name imagination task (verbal fluency), word memory task (memory/learning), common word task (reasoning), and hand movement test.

It is unique in the fact that it can be performed in a group and an average score can be obtained per age and years of education. It has been developed as screening tests of Aging Associated Cognitive Decline (AACD).

The results are considered without problem if the score is 15 after calculating by age, years of education, and gender, 11 – 14 has a possibility of AACD, less than 10 will be considered as possibility of dementia. [4]

② **How elders feel about their health and factors in daily life**

To study how the feeling of health and activities of daily life affects physical ability and cognitive function, the following investigations were made.

Currently of health : Scale of 5 from very bad to very good

Daily activities : Consists of gardening, exercise, literature/liberal arts, handicraft, music, and others

Frequency : None, 1 – 2 times a month, once a week, 2 – 3 times a week, almost daily

③ Preventative long-term care program used as basis: Effective programs extracted based on the following interventions

A 90 minute session once per month for 90 subjects, including the elderly and their families: Gather the elderly and their families, exchange information between families, and give instruction in the preventative care program: exercise, dementia prevention, stress care, eating and swallowing improvement, dietary guidance, and feedback on effectiveness.

Methods of analysis

We clarified the relationship between physical fitness test and other factors using a Pearson product-moment correlation coefficient.

3.　Result

Out of the 90 who applied for the care preventive service, there were 59 (65.6 %) who answered without any fraud, and their average age was 66.7±9.6. On the physical abilities, 11.9 % was in bad shape, scoring in the subjective physical abilities over 16, which is the cut off value. 33.3 % did not reach the average value of their age in the standing test, and 25.5 % did not reach the average value of their age in the two-step test (Figure 3-1).

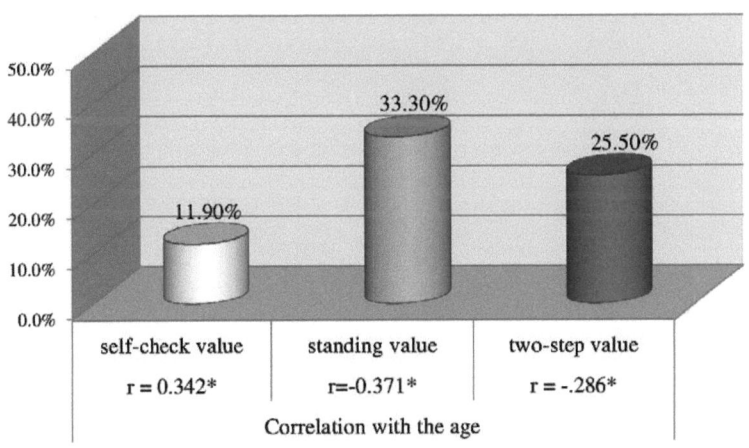

Figure 3-1. Lower ratio than the reference value of the fitness test

The relationship of age, factors in daily life, and physical ability was as the age increases, subjective physical ability declines, steps become smaller, and the ability to stand up becomes weaker (p < 0.05).

Next, the results of the Five Cog, 60 % had no problem in cognitive ability, 37.8 % was suspicion of AACD, and 2.2 % was suspicion of dementia (Figure 3-2).

The relationship between cognitive ability and physical ability was, as the two-step value becomes larger, attention (position judgment task) also became higher. Also high self-check vale resulted in high memory/learning (word memory task) (p < 0.05). No trends were seen between other factors.

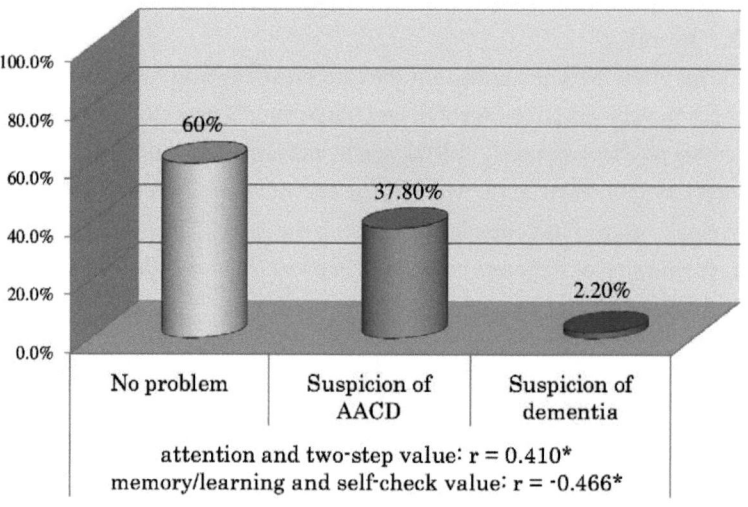

attention and two-step value: r = 0.410*
memory/learning and self-check value: r = -0.466*

Figure 3-2. Ratio of cognitive ability

As in figure 3-3, currently of health was at the bad side. A meaningful trend was when currently of health is low, the self-check value also turns out bad (p < 0.05). No other trends were seen.

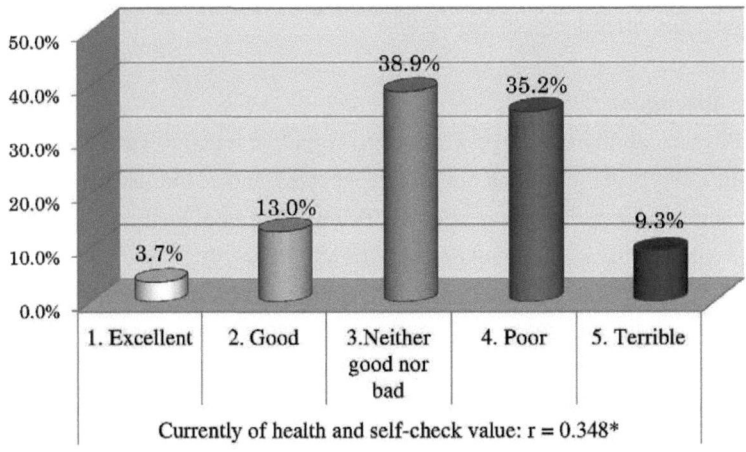

Currently of health and self-check value: r = 0.348*

Figure 3-3. Ratio of Currently of health

Next, in the daily activities, gardening was performed the most often, next was exercise then literature/liberal arts. (figure 3-4)

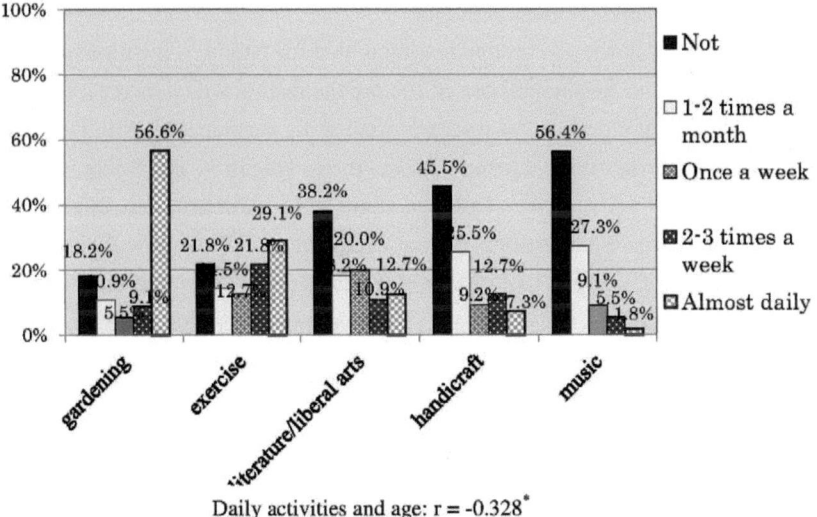

Daily activities and age: r = -0.328*

Figure 3-4. Daily activities

49

The rate of daily activities were negative against the age, as the age goes higher, activities decrease. (p < 0.05)

4. Discussion

Physical ability was largely related to cognitive function, large two-step value leads to high attention (position judgment task), and as the self-check value became higher memory/learning was also higher (word memory task). Also, self-check value was also related to currently of health.

This allows us to expect cognitive function and health will improve by continuous exercise. Past research shows elderly with short walking distance have lower cognitive function compared to long walking elders. [5] Also, it is clarified that people with active daily activities have lower risk of dementia compared to people less activities. [6]

Among the subjects of our tests, a high ratio of 44.5 % of the elders were feeling bad about their health, 21.8 % does not have habits of exercise, 14.5 % does exercise only 1 – 2 times a month. Introducing exercises to them and continuing will require effort. As reported in the second chapter of our report, letting them obtain benefit from participation and be mentally fulfilled is the key to encourage involvement of elders.

Past research shows communication with their family [7], fulfillment of social network [8], and feeling purpose of life are the factors which increases satisfaction of elders. [9] Our research predicts by participating with their family, communication will be encouraged. In this investigation, gardening was the most popular daily activity. In Japan, there were cultures of a dwarfed potted plant and Japanese traditional flower arrangement before horticultural therapy spread out, which take root in everyday life as a convenient art that can be performed indoors, and elders are very fond of it. Introducing a fond activity will promote re-recognition from memory.

From researches which study re-recognition from memory, there are two processes of recollection and familiarity during re-recognition, where recollection needs searching of detailed sentences in the step of re-recognition, but familiarity is based on senses of "seeing once before, be fond of". [10] When replaying memories, if support in decision by familiarity is made in addition of visual memory, mis-recognition of elders will be suppressed and re-recognition scores will improve. [11]

Aiming this effect, in our intervention program incorporate activities fond for the elderly. Those are in the order of familiarity, 1: gardening, 2:exercise, 3: culture, and 4:handicraft. For elders who have no habit of exercise, by incorporating exercise in familiar activities, it is thought to be more easier recognized and have stable mentality.

5. Conclusion

Physical abilities are deeply related to cognitive function, high two-step value leads to attention (position judgment task), and a high self-check value leads to high memory/learning (word memory task).

Out of the subjects of this research, a high ratio of 44.5 % feel bad about their health, 21.8 % does not have a habit of exercise, and 14.5 % exercise only 1 – 2 times a month. As a counter measure of this situation, we plan to incorporate familiar activities in our intervention for a favorable activity and improve re-recognition.

References

1) Seichi A, Hoshino Y, Doi T, et al. Development of a screening tool for risk of locomotive syndrome in the elderly: the 25-question Geriatric Locomotive Function Scale. Journal of Orthopaedic Science. 2012;17:163-172.

2) Muranaga S. Evaluation of the muscular strength of the lower extremities using the standing movement and clinical application. Journal of The Showa Medical Association. 2001;61:362-367.

3) Muranaga S, Hirano K. Development of a convenient way to predict ability to walk, using a two-step test. Journal of The Showa Medical Association. 2003;63:301-308.

4) Yatomi N. Collective cognition inspection; Five Cog. Japanese Journal of Geriatric Psychiatry. 2010;21:215-220.

5) Yaffe K, Barnes D, Nevitt M, et al. A prospective study of physical activity and cognitive decline in elderly women: women who walk. Arch Intern Med. 2001;16:1703-1708.

6) Abbott RD, White LR, Ross GW, et al. alking and dementia in physically

capable elderly men. JAMA. 2004;292:1447-1453.

7) Okamoto K. Feeling of Well-being and Family Contacts in Community Elderly Residents. Japanese Journal of Geriatrics. 2000;37:149-154.

8) Ishikawa H, Shimizu Y, Yamaguchi M. An Impact of Social Networks on Life Satisfaction among Young-old People in Japan ; Analysis of Social Networks in Terms of Area   Characteristics. Japanese Journal of Human Welfare Studies. 2009;11:49-60.

9) Okada K, Fujimoto K. A study of the factors of life worth living in community-dwelling elderly Journal of Health and Welfare Statistics. 2004;51:24-32.

10) Yonelinas AP. The nature ofrecollection and familiarity: A review of30 years ofresearch. Journal of Memory and Language. 2002;46:441-517.

11) Kunimi M, Matsukawa J. False recognition in visual short- term memory of the elderly is affected by test methods. The Japanese Journal of Psychology. 2011;82:399-405.

Chapter 4. Implementation and evaluation of a preventative care program for the elderly and family caregivers

Evaluation 1.
Exercise and cognitive function

Wakaya Fujii, Kazue Sawami, Chizuko Suishu,
Yukari Katahata, and Hirofumi Hirowatari

1. Introduction

In Chapter 3, we confirmed the relationship between exercise and cognitive function. In addition, we learned that the perception of health is low in the intervention group, and that the group also contains people with no exercise habits. In order to improve their motivation and to ensure effectiveness and continuity, an intervention program intended to incorporate familiar activities was conducted. Familiar activities were incorporated into reminiscence therapy, and a tea party was held each time in order to promote interchange between the attendees. Training focused on aerobic exercise, and the instruction on dementia prevention focused on the different actions with the right hand and the left hand, and answering a memory quiz while doing exercise and so on. All of the exercises can be performed by the family after they go home.

In order to measure the effectiveness of this, in addition to physical ability, cognitive function and daily activities, the Stages of Exercise Behaviour Change scale (SEBC), Self-Efficacy for Exercise (SEE), and the 13-item Sense of Coherence Questionnaire (SOC-13) have been added in order to compare the participants before and after and reveal their level of motivation. The previous study showed both the relationship between SEE and continuity of exercise [1], and the relationship between SOC and healthy lifestyle habits. [2-3]

In this study, the significance of scores before and after were checked in order to verify the effectiveness of intervention. Furthermore, the factors affecting SEBC and SEE and SOC were extracted to see whether they could be factors in predicting health, and the probability rate was revealed through multiple regression analysis.

2. Materials and Methods

Comparative analysis was performed before and after a six-month intervention for 90 elderly people and their families who were the subject of this study. We analyzed the effect of exercise and dementia prevention. The assessment tools are as follows.

① **Physical fitness evaluation:** Self-check sheet (The 25-question Geriatric Locomotive Function Scale), standing test, two-step test

② **Currently of health**

③ **Stages of Exercise Behaviour Change scale (SEBC):**

Stage 1: Precontemplation (Not Ready)- People are not intending to take action in the foreseeable future, and can be unaware that their behaviour is problematic.

Stage 2: Contemplation (Getting Ready)- People are beginning to recognize that their behaviour is problematic, and start to look at the pros and cons of their continued actions.

Stage 3: Preparation (Ready)- People are intending to take action in the immediate future, and may begin taking small steps toward behaviour change.

Stage 4: Action- People have made specific overt modifications in modifying their problem behaviour or in acquiring new healthy behaviours.

Stage 5: Maintenance- People have been able to sustain action for a while and are working to prevent relapse.[4]

This study scored in terms of Stage 1:1 point, Stage 2:2 point, Stage 3:3 point, Stage 4:4 point, Stage 5:5 point.

④ **Cognitive function evaluation:** Five Cog

⑤ **Frequency of the daily activities:** gardening, exercise, literature/liberal arts, handicraft, music, and others

⑥ **Self-efficacy for exercise (SEE):**

This evaluation item asks about the degree of confidence when exercising. They answer about the extent of self-confidence they have in exercise when they have physical fatigue, mental stress, are too busy, or the weather is not good in five steps.[5]

⑦ Sense of coherence (SOC):

The 13-item Sense of Coherence Questionnaire (this used the Japanese version). SOC is a concept in the salutogenic theory introduced by Antonovsky (1987). Sense of coherence (SOC) is a concept that reflects the ability to cope with stress, and is at the core of the salutogenesis theory. SOC consists of three subordinate concepts (manageability, meaningfulness and comprehensibility).[6] Each answer was selected in 7 degrees from "Never" to "Most of the time".[7-8]

Methods of analysis

The results of each evaluation scale are compared before and after using the Wilcoxon signed-rank test. Then, the factors affecting SEBC and SEE and SOC, are revealed by multiple regression analysis, and the probability that the model applies is estimated.

3. Result

The number of participants was 84 and the average age was 66.8 ± 9.8. There were 53 valid responses (63.1%).

Table 4-1. Anteroposterior comparison of scores related to the physical and cognition (N=53)

	p
self-check value	n.s.
standing value	n.s.
two-step value	0.033[*]
stages of exercise behaviour change scale	0.033[*]
cognitive function general level	0.013[*]
hand movement	n.s.
attention	n.s.
memory/learning	n.s.
visuospatial function	n.s.
verbal fluency	n.s.
reasoning	n.s.
self-efficacy for exercise	0.000[**]

comprehensibility	n.s.
manageability	0.013*
meaningfulness	n.s.

Wilcoxon signed-rank test
*Significant at the 5% level

Table 4-2. Variables affecting SEBC, SEE, and SOC ($N = 53$)

		Dependent variable					
		SEBC		SEE		SOC	
		β	P	β	P	β	P
	Age	0.552	0.001	n.s.		n.s.	
	Daily activities: literature/liberal arts	-0.357	0.018	0.461	0.012	n.s.	
	Daily activities: Exercise	n.s.		0.481	0.033	n.s.	
	Daily activities: Gardening	n.s.		0.378	0.037	0.672	0.000
	Daily activities: Music	-0.603	0.001	n.s.		n.s.	
Independent variable	Currently of health	n.s.		-0.485	0.014	-0.331	0.013
	Two-step value	n.s.		n.s.		0.313	0.038
	Standing value	n.s.		0.485	0.030	-0.417	0.006
	Self-check value	n.s.		0.568	0.029	n.s.	
	Reasoning	0.733	0.002	0.944	0.019	0.295	0.026
	Verbal fluency	-0.730	0.005	-0.687	0.023	n.s.	
	Hand movement	n.s.		0.410	0.050	n.s.	
R		0.889		0.884		0.833	
R-squared		0.791		0.782		0.694	
Adjusted R-squared		0.657		0.632		0.610	

Multiple regression analysis: backward elimination method.
Results of the analysis are shown on the table with standard partial regression coefficient (β), contribution ratio (R^2) and conformance of model (adjusted R^2). The β value shows the size of the impact of each independent variable on the dependent variable (SEBC, SEE, SOC), where the larger the β value the greater the impact on the dependent variant. Note that the table only includes β values with a significant variation.

As shown in Table 4-1, in terms of physical ability, the two-step value was significantly improved, and in terms of motivation the stages of exercise behavior change scale was improved. The total level was also improved in regard to cognitive functionality. In addition, self-efficacy for exercise and SOC of manageability were improved ($p < 0.05$).

Following this, multiple regression analysis clarified what affects the SEBC and SEE and SOC. The factors that affect the SEBC are age, literature/liberal arts activities, music activities, reasoning ability, and verbal fluency. Factors that affect SEE are literature/liberal arts activities, music activities, gardening, the perception of one's current health, standing value, self-check value, reasoning ability, and verbal fluency. Factors that affect SOC were gardening, the perception of one's current health, two-step value, standing value and reasoning ability ($p < 0.05$). There is a probability that all of these models apply (adjusted $R^2 > 0.6$).

4. Discussion

By comparing the data before and after the intervention, we can see that the sub-scale of exercise, cognition, behavior modification, self-efficacy, and sense of coherence were significantly improved, which proves that the new care preventive program is effective. In addition, the factors influencing the SEBC and SEE and SOC were revealed.

Factors affecting SEBC are age, and literature/liberal arts activities and music activities from among daily activities. We can see that everyday activities are highly influential in SEE and SOC, and the importance of familiar activities was also revealed. In our care preventive intervention, we included familiar activities, and these are believed to be effective factors. Furthermore, reasoning ability and verbal fluency skills are considered to be highly related, and the ability to predict thinking as part of cognitive function was found to be required for behavior.

Factors affecting SEE, were found to be literature/liberal arts activities, music activities, and gardening as part of daily activities, physical activities, the perception of one's current health, self-check value and standing value. Physical functions also affected SOC, and good circulation through the synergistic effects is expected as part of this functional training. In terms of cognitive abilities, the same factors that affect SEBC, such as reasoning ability and verbal fluency were significantly influential and the training of these two abilities was found to be essential.

Factors affecting SOC were gardening from among everyday activities, physical activities, the perception of one's current health, two-step value, standing value, and reasoning ability as part of cognition. It was revealed that a sense of stability could be achieved through the feeling of something as consistent or understanding something through familiar activities or the perception of one's health and the ability to predict. For all of these models, the probability that they apply and may become a factor to predict the health is high.

For the familiar activities affecting all items, activating the various functions has been found to be effective. Those who engage in familiar activities, those who can achieve relaxation through gardening and music[9-10], and can improve their mental health through paintings[11] have been reported to maintain neuropsychological functions than those who do not. [12]

Similarly, the result of this study shows that synergistic effects, combining cognitive training and exercise, and familiar activities, have been found to be more effective.

5. Conclusion

We have confirmed that the new care preventive program which combines familiar activities and exercise can lead to significant improvements in exercise, cognition, behavior modification, self-efficacy, and sense of coherence. Familiar activities, reasoning ability and verbal fluency are factors that affect SEBC, and these are the same factors as for SEE. The exercise function also affects SEE. Factors affecting SOC are familiar activities, the perception of one's current health, exercise function and reasoning ability.

Combining familiar activities, exercise and recognition training revealed to be effective. There is a high probability that these models apply and that they may become factors for predicting health.

References
1) Maeba K, Takenaka K. Effects of Efficacy-Enhancing Interventions to Exercise Maintenance among Older Adults−A Preliminary Examination Using

a Meta-Analysis —. Japanese Journal of Behavioral Medicine. 2012;18:36-40.

2) Sagara T, Hitomi Y, Kambayashi Y, et al. Common risk factors for changes in body weight
   and psychological well-being in Japanese male middle-aged workers. Environ Health Prev Med. 2009;14:319–327.

3) Shintani N, Takao F, Nakamura Y, et al. A study on the lifestyle or job related factors causing the mental and physical complaints and enforcing the sense of coherence. The Bulletin of Department of Health and Social Services, Hiroshima International University. 2008;4:111-121.

4) Oka K. Reliability and validity of the stages of change for exercise behavior scale among
   middle-aged adults. Japanese Journal of Health Promotion. 2003;5:15-22.

5) Oka K. Stages of change for exercise behavior and self-efficacy for exercise among middle-aged adults. Nihon Koshu Eisei Zasshi. 2003;50:208-215.

6) Togari T, Yamazaki Y, Nakayama K, et al. Development of a short version of the sense of coherence scale for population survey. J Epidemiol Community Health. 2007;61:921–922.

7) Antonovsky A. Unraveling the Mystery of Health: How People Manage Stress and Stay Well [Kenko-no-nazo-wo-toku] Trans Yamazaki Y, Yoshii K. Tokyo: Yushindo Kobunsha; 1987.

8) Yamazaki Y. Sakano J, and Togari T. Stress coping abilities SOC. Yushindo Kobunsha. Tokyo. 2008; 3-24.

9) Lee MS, Park BJ, Lee J, et al. Physiological relaxation induced by horticultural activity: transplanting work using flowering plants. Journal of Physiological Anthropology. 2013;32:1-5.

10) kotake N, Nakamura K, Takahashi Y. Research on the Relaxation Effect of Music Therapy. Journal of the Faculty of Nursing and Nutrition Siebold University of Nagasaki. 2005;5:1-10.

11) Kawakubo E, Uchida Y, Koizumi M. "Art Therapy" Implementation and Evaluation in Older Persons with Dementia. The Kitakanto Medical Journal. 2011;61:499-508.

12) Fratiglioni L, Paillard BS, Winblad B. An active and socially integrated lifestyle in late life may protect against dementia. The Lancet Neurology. 2004;3:343-353.

Evaluation 2.
Psychological effects

Kazue Sawami, Wakaya Fujii, Chizuko Suishu,
Katahata Yukari, and Hirofumi Hirowatari

1. Introduction

As previously described, the number of elderly people play a role of family caregivers in Japan, and in most cases, elderly woman is taking care of her husband or people around 60 years old are taking care of their parents around 80 to 90 years old. Because of these circumstances, aged caregivers have few chances to gain useful information about an elderly care. By considering these backgrounds, it is crucial for Japanese society to offer a support for the family caregivers or elderly people who care older people.

Prior research has shown that the direct communication among family caregivers cultivates a better understanding on nursing skills and brings an opportunity for them to feel similar emotions with each other and builds a sense of solidarity, and hence it forms positive emotion within caregivers[1].

In this research, elderly people and their family members were gathered and they were given the information related to the nursing, and encouraged to interact with each other. The aim of this research is to reveal the effect of this intervention to build the effective strategy on elderly care of future Japanese society. There is also a report that the sense of burden in family caregivers can cause depression[2] and decreased Health-Related Quality Of Life (HRQOL)[3]. Therefore, the feeling scale and HRQOL of the intervention group and control group were compared before and after the intervention for the prevention of the elderly care.

2. Materials and Methods

Research participants are the same as Evaluation 1. In this research, HRQOL and feeling of 84 people in the intervention group and 100 people in the control group were examined before and after the intervention for the prevention of the elderly care.

The assessment methods that were uses in this research are as follows:

① Measurement of psychological reaction to stress: Profile of Mood States - Brief form (POMS) Japanese version

This uses six scales, "tension-anxiety," "depression-dejection," "anger-hostility," "fatigue-inertia," "vigor-activity," and "confusion-bewilderment," to measure the state of feelings and emotions. There are a total of 30 question items, and subjects respond whether they experienced each item in the preceding week on a 5-level scale ranging from "not at all" to "very much."

② Health-related quality of life (QOL) measurement: WHO Quality of Life 26 (WHO-QOL26) Japanese version

This is composed of 24 times that evaluate the four areas of QOL, the physical area, the psychological area, social relations, and the environmental area, as well as two items that evaluate overall QOL, for a total of 26 items. Subjects respond to 26 items about how they felt in the past two weeks and how satisfied they were in the past two weeks on a 5-level scale: "not at all," "just a little," "somewhat," "very much," and "extremely."

③ Satisfaction with the Program Conducted

Subjects answer how satisfied they were after the intervention on a 10-level scale from "dissatisfied" to "very satisfied."

Methods of analysis

The Wilcoxon signed-rank test was used to examine the effect of intervention on participants in the intervention group before and after the intervention. Results of the intervention group and control group were investigated by the analysis of variance (ANOVA) after that.

3. Result

The valid responses were collected from 52 people (61.9%) in the intervention group which was formed with the same participants from the Evaluation 1 while the valid answers were collected from 72 out of 100 people (72.0%) in the control group. The average age of the participants in the control group was 65.5 ± 4.7.

Table 4-3. Before-and-after survey on QOL and POMS of the intervention group $(N = 52)$

Test items		p
POMS	Tension-anxiety	0.000**
	Depression-dejection	0.000**
	Anger-hostility	n.s.
	Fatigue-inertia	0.002**
	Vigor-activity	0.000**
	Confusion-bewilderment	0.007**
WHO-QOL26	Overall	0.007**
	Physical	0.000**
	Psychological	0.000**
	Social	0.045*
	Environmental	n.s.

Wilcoxon signed-rank test
*Significant at the 5% level, **Significant at the 1% level.

As for the results of before-and-after survey on intervention group by the Wilcoxon signed-rank test that are shown in table 4-3, statistically significant increases were found in overall, physical, psychological (p < 0.01) and social domain (p < 0.05) of QOL. With the Profile of Mood States (POMS), a significant decrease in tension-anxiety, depression- dejection, fatigue-inertia, confusion-bewilderment and significant increase in vigor-activity (p < 0.01) were observed.

Subsequently, a significant difference between the results of the before-and-after survey on control group and intervention group were revealed by the analysis of variance.

As shown in table 4-4, before the intervention, significantly lower Overall-QOL and Psychological-QOL were observed in the intervention group.

However, after the intervention, the Psychological-QOL has significantly increased and surpassed the rate of Psychological-QOL of control group (p < 0.05).

Table 4-4. Comparison of WHO-QOL26 & POMS test items before and after intervention (N= 124)

Test items		Group	Before intervention				After intervention			
			Descriptive statistics		Analysis of variance		Descriptive statistics		Analysis of variance	
			mean	S.D.	F	p	mean	S.D.	F	p
WHO-QOL26	Overall	intervention	3.312	0.593	6.857	0.010[*]	3.591	0.547	0.003	0.955
		control	3.570	0.565			3.597	0.502		
	Physical	intervention	3.692	0.634	0.373	0.542	3.969	0.448	12.298	0.001[**]
		control	3.757	0.614			3.695	0.390		
	Psychological	intervention	3.420	0.596	8.367	0.004[**]	3.785	0.486	4.719	0.032[*]
		control	3.686	0.489			3.603	0.411		
	Social	intervention	3.492	0.629	0.985	0.323	3.671	0.516	0.605	0.438
		control	3.405	0.406			3.604	0.416		
	Environmental	intervention	3.523	0.536	2.598	0.109	3.548	0.515	3.352	0.070
		control	3.663	0.485			3.706	0.414		
POMS	Tension-anxiety	intervention	5.592	4.364	15.218	0.000[**]	3.741	3.000	1.459	0.229
		control	3.407	2.649			4.319	2.386		
	Depression-dejection	intervention	3.684	3.882	6.796	0.010[*]	2.655	2.432	0.223	0.638
		control	2.288	2.738			2.449	2.465		
	Anger-hostility	intervention	2.895	3.353	6.844	0.010[*]	2.655	2.468	0.073	0.787
		control	1.675	2.417			2.768	2.230		
	Vigor-activity	intervention	7.803	3.936	15.908	0.000[**]	10.000	3.709	0.078	0.780
		control	10.225	3.649			10.188	3.844		
	Fatigue-inertia	intervention	5.184	4.583	14.508	0.000[**]	4.103	3.655	0.113	0.738
		control	2.838	2.983			3.913	2.732		
	Confusion-bewilderment	intervention	5.579	3.360	4.837	0.029[*]	4.345	2.482	1.332	0.251
		control	4.525	2.595			4.826	2.216		

Analysis of variance

S.D.: standard deviation

By comparing the results of POMS, although tension-anxiety, depression-dejection, anger-hostility, fatigue-inertia and confusion-bewilderment were significantly higher and vigor-activity was significantly lower with the caregivers and their old parents in the intervention group before the intervention, people in the intervention group have enhanced their mood after the intervention, and the rate of those factors were no longer different from that of control group.

Through the entire care prevention program, the activities with high degree of satisfaction from the participants were examined. The average satisfaction degree in Swedish massage was 9.93, prevention activities on dementia was 9.87, physical activity was 9.87, music therapy was 9.80 (Maximum rate was 10.0).

4. Discussion

Tension-anxiety, depression-dejection, anger-hostility, fatigue-inertia and confusion-bewilderment were significantly higher and vigor-activity was significantly lower with the elderly people and their family members in intervention group if compare with the people in the control group. It is assumed that those people felt nervous when they met with complete strangers and could not imagine what kind of intervention they will receive. As described in previous chapter, the health status was significantly lower with people in intervention group. It is expected that those conditions affected their QOL and feeling. It can be also said that their tiredness and perplexity have resulted their health status.

The highest degree of satisfaction was observed in Swedish massage which is mainly for the stress prevention. Swedish massage is the soft touch massage that has a relaxing effect. It is possible that the elderly people and their family members have made a mentally comfortable communication by massaging with each other. There is no custom of making physical contact with people in close relationship such as shaking hand or hugging each other in Japan, particularly among the elderly people. Though, the result of high degree of satisfaction in this research has revealed the effectiveness of the physical contact. It is an effective and useful method for elderly people to reduce stress at home since the elderly people have few chance of making physical contact other than their family members.

Since Swedish massage is expected to have positive physical effect and

64

physiological effect[4-6], if participants of the research continue this activity at home, they can expect to have health improvement.

Prevention activities on dementia and physical activity which were examined their effectiveness at Evaluation 1 marked high degree of satisfaction next to Swedish massage. Music therapy is quite a familiar activity for many participants and was examined its effectiveness in Chapter.3.

These interventions lowered tension-anxiety, depression-dejection, fatigue-inertia and confusion-bewilderment significantly, and raised vigor-activity in mental states of participants. Tension-easing from the promotion of communication among the participants, getting healthy by improving physical condition with physical activity, relieving the concern by gaining information about nursing and health and rise in vigor-activity by involving their familiar activity can be considered as causes of these changes.

As of QOL, overall, physical, psychological, social-QOL had significantly increased. By considering the increase in social-QOL, these change occurred not only because of the physical activity and stress prevention but also caused by the communication activity.

If compare the mental states of participants in intervention group and control group before the intervention, overall mental states of participants in intervention group were lower than that of control group, particularly psychological-QOL was significantly lower. After the intervention, overall mental states of participants in intervention group have increased; especially physical-QOL has increased dramatically. These changes were the result of continuity of recommended activities. The most variable finding of this research was that the participants could proactively adopt the recommended activities.

The subject of future research is how to maintain the recommended activities and self-efficacy is said to be the important factor to keep up these activities[7-8] and those factors which effect on self-efficacy and adoption of activity were revealed in Evaluation 1. Those factors are familiar activity, health status, physical condition, thinking ability and linguistic ability. By offering training related to those factors on participants, maintainability in self-efficacy and adopted activity is excepted to be revealed in longitudinal research.

5. Conclusion

Those elderly people and their family members who participated in this research were feeling uneasy, nervous, tired and inactive, and their psychological-QOL was lower before the intervention for the prevention of the elderly care. These circumstances seemed to indicate the influence of the lower health state of the elderly people and tiredness of family caregivers. Among the intervention for the stress prevention, Swedish massage has marked the highest degree of satisfaction and this result indicated the importance of physical contact among the elderly people and family caregivers.

After the intervention, both QOL and feeling have improved significantly. Particularly, the degree of physical-QOL of participants in intervention group was outstanding and has surpassed that of participants in the control group. These changes were the result of continuity of recommended activities which participants adopted in their daily life.

As a subject of future research, the probability of continuing the adopted activities is expected to be revealed in longitudinal research.

References

1) Suganuma M, Nitta S. Literature Review of Interventions for Family Caregivers of the Elderly with Dementia. Journal of Japan Academy of Gerontological Nursing. 2012;17:74-82.

2) Yates ME, Tennstedt S, Chang B. Contributors to and mediators of psychological well-being for informal caregivers. Journal of Gerontology: Psychological Sciences. 1999;54B:12–22.

3) Miyashita M, Sakai M, Iitsuka H, et al. Burdens to Family Members in Home Care and Related QOL Factors. Journal of the Japanese Association of Rural Medicine. 2006;54:767-773.

4) Rapaport MH, Schettler P, Bresee C. A Preliminary Study of the Effects of a Single Session of Swedish Massage on Hypothalamic–Pituitary–Adrenal and Immune Function in Normal Individuals. The Journal of Alternative and Complementary Medicine. 2010;16:1079-1088.

5) Kaye AD, Kaye AJ, Swinford J, et al. The Effect of Deep-Tissue Massage Therapy on Blood Pressure and Heart Rate. The Journal of Alternative and Complementary Medicine. 2008;14: 125-128.

6) Vahedian-Azimi A, Ebadi A, Jafarabadi MA, et al. Effect of Massage Therapy on Vital Signs and GCS Scores of ICU Patients: A Randomized Controlled Clinical Trial. Trauma Monthly. 2014;19:19-25.
7) Inaba Y, Obuchi S, Arai T, et al. Effects of exercise intervention on exercise behavior in community-dwelling elderly subjects: A randomized controlled trial. Japanese Journal of Geriatrics. 2013;50:788-796.
8) Takai I. A study of factors influenced by self-efficacy for exercise among community- dwelling elderly men in urban areas. Japanese Journal of Geriatrics. 2012;49:740-745.

Acknowledgments

We would like to thank all the elderly people and their families for participating in the preventative care project. We also appreciate the full cooperation from the staff of Japan Agricultural Cooperatives Nishimino who agreed with the purpose of this research and helped us to plan, recruit the participants, communicate, arrange the venue, and do the reception. We thank Mr. Ban, Mrs. Takagi, Kitamura and all other staff from our heart.

We also thank Professor Sugiura, managing executive Mr. Okazaki and all other staff from Japan health recreation society for cooperating in the class for the elderly people and their families.

Epilog

We have carried out this study laying emphasis on improving quality of life for elderly people and their families through long-term preventative care programs. By establishing a respondents' participation engagement structure, we have considered and implemented an appropriate intervention and elicited future objectives from the results.

Thus far, long-term preventative care programs were not always implemented strategically. In order for preventative methods to pervade among the elderly and their families, programs require a thorough strategy. Therefore, related academic institutions and private organizations need to address overall long-term preventative care projects in collaboration and enhance support for the elderly and their families. Although we have two universities, one academic community and one public organization as our foundation, we plan to expand our regional partnership and to pursue the support required for the present situation of the elderly in the region.

In this study, we have demonstrated causal correlations between physical function, cognitive function, and other factors that affect quality of life. By forecasting each person's future based on the findings, we seek to provide individualized preventative care programs and to improve subjects' benefits.

Authors
Kazue Sawami
   Department of Gerontological Nursing, Nara Medical University
Wakaya Fujii
   Department of Occupational therapy, Gifu Junior College Of Health Science
Chizuko Suishu
   Department of Gerontological Nursing, Nara Medical University
Yukari Katahata
   Department of Gerontological Nursing, Nara Medical University
Hirofumi Hirowatari
   Department of Occupational therapy, Gifu Junior College Of Health Science
Naoko Morisaki

Department of Gerontological Nursing, University of KinDAI Himeji

Hidekazu Koufuku
Department of Occupational therapy, University of Tokyo Health Sciences

Hiroko Miura
Department of Dentistry, National Institute of Public Health

Sonomi Hattori
Department of Gerontological Nursing, Wakayama Medical University

Tomoko Ishitani
Department of Gerontological Nursing, Wakayama Medical University

Xiao-Jing Li
Faculty of Nursing, Shandong University

Feng-Lan Lou
Faculty of Nursing, Shandong University

Correspondence address: Kazue Sawami
Department of Gerontological Nursing, Nara Medical University
840 Shijo-cho, Kashihara, Nara JAPAN
Tel: 81-744-22-3051
E-mail: k-sawami@tius-hs.jp

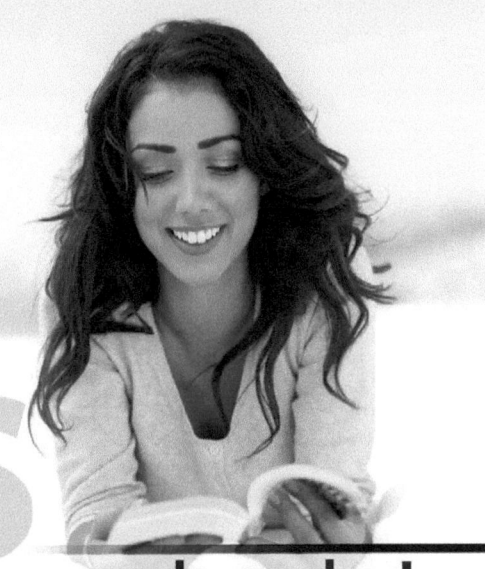
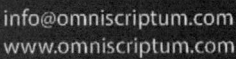
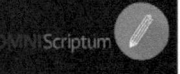

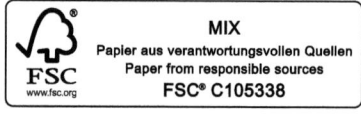

Printed by Books on Demand GmbH, Norderstedt / Germany